CARERS PERCEIVED

CARERS PERCEIVED
Policy and practice in informal care

JULIA TWIGG AND
KARL ATKIN

OPEN UNIVERSITY PRESS
Buckingham · Philadelphia

Open University Press
Celtic Court
22 Ballmoor
Buckingham
MK18 1XW

and
1900 Frost Road, Suite 101
Bristol, PA 19007, USA

First Published 1994

A catalogue record of this book is available from the British Library

ISBN 0 335 19111 8 (pb) 0 335 19112 6 (hb)

Library of Congress Cataloging-in-Publication Data
Twigg, Julia.
Carers perceived: policy and practice in informal care / Julia Twigg and Karl Atkin.
p. cm.
Includes bibliographical references and index.
ISBN 0-335-19112-6 (hardback) ISBN 0-335-19111-8 (pbk.)
1. Caregivers—Great Britain. 2. Social services—Great Britain.
3. Health services—Great Britain. I. Atkin, Karl. II. Title.
HV248.T95 1993
362.1'0425—dc20 93-15944
CIP

Typeset by Best-set Typesetter Ltd, Hong Kong
Printed in Great Britain by Biddles Limited, Guildford and Kings Lynn

CONTENTS

ACKNOWLEDGEMENTS

The research that underpins the book was commissioned by the Department of Health, and we are grateful for the space they gave us to develop the work further. Our thanks go to Jenny Griffin, Sue Moylan, Madeleine Simms and Ruth Chadwick of the Research Management Division. Particular thanks are due to Christina Perring who was involved in the fieldwork and early stages of the analysis. Most of all, our thanks must go to our colleagues at the Social Policy Research Unit, University of York, particularly Gillian Parker, Michael Hirst and Jan Rollings. Lorna Foster and Jenny Bowes gave invaluable help in the final stages of preparing the book. Last, Julia Twigg would like to record a personal intellectual debt to Bleddyn Davies, and more distantly to David Martin.

Chapter 1 INFORMAL CARE

Carers are no longer the Cinderellas of social policy. One of the striking developments of the last decade has been the increasing reference to carers in public policy documents. Government pronouncements in relation to the new community care consistently refer to 'users and carers'. Conferences are held to discuss their needs, and guidance issued as to their support. Politicians find it expedient to refer to carers in their speeches. They are seen as a worthy focus for charitable activity – one linked to the common experiences of many and untainted by associations with the undeserving. Carers have moved out of the shadows into the policy arena.

Despite this greater visibility of carers in the policy debate, policy itself has not engaged in any sustained way with their incorporation, remaining undeveloped and seldom going beyond bland statements of the importance of supporting carers. But which carers, in what ways, and to what ends, are rarely discussed. Despite their virtues and the acknowledged centrality of the carer issue, there has been little in the way of strategic thinking on the subject among policymakers and planners.

This lack of theorizing about the relationship between carers and services has found its parallel in the academic literature. As a result of the explosion of research on caring that has taken place over the last decade (Parker 1990a; Twigg 1992), we now have a relatively good understanding of the nature of caring – its origins, incidence, patterns and experiences. We also have some understanding from surveys and qualitative studies of the sorts of help that carers say they would like, and of the role of specific, usually small-scale, schemes in their support. What we do *not* have is a well-based understanding of how carers fit into the service system, and of how their needs are, and are not, incorporated into the practice of mainstream service providers. Which carers get help and why? What assumptions are made about different carers, and how do these mediate the responses to them that are seen as appropriate and legitimate? How are carers perceived? The academic literature until now has not addressed these questions. We have also lacked theoretical models for the relationship between carers and service provision. How *should* agencies respond to carers? What factors should determine provision? What are the implications of targeting? Carers cannot be seen in isolation from the rest of service provision, and their needs and interests have to be placed within a wider context. What mechanisms do we have for this? How can we balance the interests of the carer and the cared for?

These are the questions that are explored in this book. In addressing them, we map a new intellectual territory in regard to carers, one that explores their position within the service system. The account that we give, however, has a wider significance than simply the subject of carers. Carers expose, sometimes in more acute forms, issues that are general within public policy, and many of the points that we shall make and the conceptual structures we shall suggest in this book are as relevant to the situation of clients and patients as of carers. Caring needs to be seen within that wider context.

In this opening chapter, we concentrate on caring itself, exploring the intellectual sources of the current debate and the different strands of discussion. We then turn to the concept of caring, and the elements that make up the experience. Finally, we examine the implications for policy and for analysis of the fact that caring takes place in a relationship in which the cared-for person as well as the carer has needs and interests.

The strands in the debate

The first of the strands in the debate has been the changing academic understanding of kinship obligation. During the 1950s and 1960s, sociological understanding of the family was dominated by a Parsonian functionalism that emphasized the structural affinities between the modern nuclear family and the conditions of industrial or capitalist production. The *family* was interpreted narrowly in terms of the nuclear *household* with its functional specialism, and little or no attention was paid to wider kinship obligations, which were assumed to have withered away with the rise of modern industrial society. Young and Wilmott's famous study of the East End (1957), which did chart important transfers of support between households and generations particularly between women, was seen as providing a dramatic contrast to the dominant account, but one that described an enclave of survival rather than a reality that could be considered to be widely current. As a result, caring as we understand it now was absent from the analytic agenda: an academic subject that simply did not exist. This found its echo in commonly expressed moralistic views that asserted that people no longer cared for their parents or family in the way that they had in the past.

This consensus began to break up in the late 1970s and 1980s primarily under the impact of feminism. Feminism challenged the traditional sociology of the family, exploding its complacency, and exposing its normative biases and unexplored assumptions about the role of women. With the growing realization in the 1980s of the variety of household forms also came a more sophisticated understanding of the distinction between household and family, which freed the analysis of family obligation from its earlier conceptual strait-jacket. Interest in kinship obligation in providing care was strengthened and deepened by a growing historical literature on the family, exemplified in the work of Anderson,

Laslett and the Cambridge Group. This disrupted earlier easy assumptions about the past as a golden age of family support (Anderson 1971, 1980; Laslett 1972, 1977; Smith 1984; Thomson 1991).

Qureshi and Walker's analysis of the family care of older people established the normative priorities governing who gives care in the family; and Finch and Mason have taken the sociological analysis of obligation a step further in their detailed exploration of the ways in which kinship rules are negotiated in concrete situations (Finch 1989; Qureshi and Walker 1989; Finch and Mason 1993). As a result we now have a new understanding of how family obligations operate; and this change in academic understanding has been influential in the way the debate on informal care has developed. Although politicians and members of the public still occasionally talk of the family failing in its duty, this is not how the debate on informal care is now structured. Qureshi and Walker (1989: 2) express the new orthodoxy when they comment:

> contrary to the views strongly held by some politicians there is no *evidence* whatsoever of a significant unwillingness to care on the part of families. Indeed we were struck, first by the universal nature of the acceptance of their primary role in the provision of care for elderly relatives (particularly by female kin) and, second, by the tremendous normative pressure on them to do so. (original emphasis)

The second influential strand in the debate has been feminism. The feminist critique of community care emerged in the late 1970s and early 1980s, associated with the work of Finch and Groves, Graham, Wilson and others (Land 1978; Finch and Groves 1980, 1983; Wilson 1982; Graham 1983, 1991; Ungerson 1983, 1987; Land and Rose 1985; Dalley 1988; Baldwin and Twigg 1991). Its origins lay in the continuation and extension of feminist debates concerning childcare, the role of women's unpaid labour and the significance of the family in public policy. Feminists exposed the ways in which social policy contained an implicit family policy in which the position of women was assumed and unchallenged. Particular concern was expressed at the growing emphasis in public policy on community care (Wilson 1982), and its implications for informal carers, perceived to be predominantly women. Women were seen as the new reserve army of – this time – unpaid labour. The sense of injustice arising from the unequal burden of caring borne by women found particular focus in the equal opportunity issues raised by the failure to extend Invalid Care Allowance (ICA) to married women (Finch and Groves 1980). Caring was seen to block access to socially valued market place resources, thereby perpetuating powerlessness (Hooyman 1990). Finally, the feminist analysis was not just concerned with labour but also with love, and feminists such as Graham (1983) argued that women internalize a self-identity around caring in ways that mean they set their priorities in terms of the needs of others, devaluing their own.

The discovery, in the wake of the 1985 *GHS* data (Green 1988), of unexpected numbers of male carers disrupted the earlier assumption that caring was almost exclusively a women's issue. Further analysis of the data, however, revealed that the majority of these male carers were spouses and/or that they were involved in the lighter end of caregiving (Parker and Lawton 1990a, 1990b;

Parker 1992). Intergenerational care involving long hours and intimate personal care was still heavily gendered. The *GHS* figures and other work (Parker 1992) did, however, make visible the extent to which caring is carried out in spouse relations, redressing the earlier bias, in part created by the personal concerns of feminists, towards seeing carers solely as daughters and daughters-in-law. These changes in the understanding of caring did not invalidate the feminist critique, which remains the single most sophisticated body of theorizing in the field, though they did suggest that additional elements needed to be incorporated into it.

More recently the feminist analysis of informal care has itself begun to change, moving away from what Graham (1991) describes as the 'consensus and continuity' that was a hallmark of the earlier period. Two developments have been particularly significant. The first is the growing integration of the analysis of informal care with that of paid caring work, exemplified in the work of Graham on paid domestic labour and Ungerson on payment for caring (Graham 1991; Ungerson and Baldock 1991; Ungerson, forthcoming). The impulse for this shift comes from the feminist concern to break down the analytic division of public/private and explore how women's caring work in each sphere structures aspects of the other. The second development has arisen out of wider debates within feminist theory that have exposed the degree to which earlier feminist analysis was based on the experiences of white, middle-class women, excluding those of black, working-class women whose experiences were treated as special and separate. The new analysis of caring has attempted to show the ways in which women can be subject to different forms of oppression of which gender is only one (Graham 1991). Williams (1989) has argued in another context how social policy has failed to incorporate the dimensions of class, race (and gender).

Allied to these more theoretical arguments has been a body of empirical work – sometimes explicitly feminist in inspiration but not always – that described the impact of caring. Such work explored the daily grind of care-giving and the heavy costs it imposes – emotional, physical and financial (Nissel and Bonnerjea 1982; Glendinning 1983, 1992; Baldwin 1985; Wright 1986; Parker 1993). This perception was reinforced by the emergence in the 1980s of the carer lobby led by what is now the Carers National Association, creating an effective focus for pressure group politics and helping to push the carer issue onto the policy agenda. Out of this has developed an approach that emphasizes the ways in which caring disrupts normal life, imposing special burdens that need to be alleviated. Carers in this tradition are not perceived so much as women or families, but as people whose lives have been significantly disrupted by caring, and this focus gives a slightly different emphasis to the debate, which centres around a discourse of justice and of individual 'need' in which certain burdens are seen to be beyond normal expectations, calling for public intervention and support.

The literature on burden and stress has been a large one, particularly in the United States. Although it has included ethnographic and sociological accounts of the burden of care, it has been dominated by psychological methodology. The impetus behind the pursuit of measures of stress has partly been one of establishing in concrete and visible form the personal costs of caring, and partly developing objective measures of the impact of different interventions. More recently the approach has been subject to criticism. Measures of burden and stress have been presented as chimeras whose pursuit yields increasingly diminishing returns (Zarit 1989). Stress or burden have been reified, pursued in ways that are detached either from how people cope with their lives or the policy issues posed by caring. Criticism of the emphasis on burden also arises from academics and lobbyists who argue that this is not how many carers perceive their situations, and that the language is pathologizing.

Coming from a very different direction has been the influence particularly in the 1980s of the New Right and its critique of the welfare state (Anderson *et al.* 1981; Flynne 1989). In general, writers in this tradition have not explicitly engaged with the issue of informal care, though the subject is present obliquely in the emphasis on personal responsibility for welfare and the promotion of conservative family values that reassert the primacy of the traditional family, in the sense of the married couple with children, where the wife is dependent and the husband the primary breadwinner and, in some degree, the source of moral authority. Although such writing contains a general endorsement of family ties and responsibilities (Anderson and Dawson 1986), its essentially individualistic and male focus, deriving from its neo-liberal roots, means that it does not go beyond the nuclear family, and the direct support of elderly or disabled people does not form a central theme in this account. New Right thinkers, when they have considered the question, tend to concentrate on issues of funding, exploring, for example, the release of equity in housing or the empowerment of elderly people by vouchers or consumerism (Laing 1991; Oldman 1991). There were some muted references in the 1980s to the 'liable relatives' tradition of the Poor Law, whereby children were financially liable for the support of their parents, but these were not take further.

The principal impact of New Right ideas arose less in relation to ideas of family obligation than in response to fears of the fiscal crisis that, it was argued, threatened societies with advanced welfare states. The burden of taxation and the proportion of GNP distributed through the state were regarded as barriers to economic health as well as being undesirable in themselves. If these burdens were to be shifted – particularly in the context of rising numbers of elderly people – an alternative source of help would need to be identified: informal care was the obvious one. At first this found expression in assertions that the resources of the informal sector were underutilized and that there were untapped sources of help to be found in the 'community' and the voluntary sector. Anxieties were expressed lest services drive out family care. No evidence was found to support either of these propositions, and the debate shifted away from these supposed potentialities towards the need to support carers as the cheapest means of supporting elderly and disabled people. This bring us to the fifth theme in the debate: that of the rationalization of community care.

Care in the community has been the dominant theme of government policy since the 1960s. Implementation accelerated in the 1980s, partly associated with the hospital closure programme, but also as a result of renewed Government commitment to the policy. Community care was regarded as the best form of care and, more equivocally, as the most cost-effective form of care. Pressure to develop more effective provision also came from the massive expansion of private residential care funded by social security payments. The desire to cap this budget and remove the perverse incentives created by it (Audit Commission 1986) produced a new agenda for community care. This was, however, overtaken by developments in the NHS, particularly the institution of the internal market, to which community care was increasingly seen as an adjunct.

The 1980s had been a period of declining net resources in social services – although there has been a rise in resources, costs have risen at a faster rate (Bebbington and Kelly 1992) – and the New Managerialism (Stewart 1986), which emphasized specificity of objectives, cost-effectiveness and value for money audit, was in part a response to this and the consequent need to rationalize community care. In this, carers were seen as a resource whose 'price' to social care agencies was very low: they only needed to put in small amounts of formal resources to ensure extensive inputs from the informal sector. Supporting carers represented a highly cost-effective strategy, a point that was often emphasized in attempts to justify funding. The argument was rarely expressed in its most naked form, whereby the *only* reason to alleviate the circumstances of a carer was in order to ensure that he or she continued to give care; but in its more benign versions, which blurred the focus of the intervention somewhat, it was widely influential.

The most recent influence in the debate has been an increasingly powerful critique put forward by the disability lobby. This centres on work that emphasizes the ways in which disability is socially constructed, and repudiates the oppression inherent in the medical model or the lay emphasis on disability as personal tragedy (Oliver 1990; Morris 1991). The social creation of disability and of caring are seen as linked: 'All the factors which transform an impairment into a disability also tend to transform family members and friends into informal carers' (Parker 1992: 17). Out of these perceptions has developed a critique of the debate on informal care, which argues that policy should not endorse dependence through an emphasis on supporting carers, but underwrite the independence of the disabled people they 'care' for. People with disabilities should be able to make and have personal and family relationships, but these should not become the basis of caring. The recent emphasis on the needs of carers, in this view, diverts attention and resources from what is the real issue, that of the support of disabled people. Morris (1991), in particular, criticizes the earlier feminist work for its failure to incorporate the subjective experiences of the recipients of care – and this in a literature that emphasizes how the personal is political. Many of the people being cared for are women, a fact rarely addressed in the feminist analysis; and Morris suggests that feminism constitutes its subject – women – in a way that excludes disabled women.

These then are the main ways in which the debate around caring has been structured. We now turn to more particular issues, exploring the categorization of carers and the concept of caring employed in this study.

The categorization of carers: the generic approach

There are three main ways in which carers have been categorized in studies: in terms of features of themselves (child carers, male carers), in terms of features of the cared-for person (carers of stroke victims, of older people), and in terms of their relationship (spouse carers, non-kin carers). Most work has limited itself in terms of one and sometimes two of these dimensions. Thus Lewis and Meredith (1988) studied women caring for their mothers; Levin and her colleagues (1989) people caring for an older person with dementia; and Parker (1993) non-elderly spouse carers of physically disabled people. This book, by contrast, is not confined to a particular category of carer. Instead, we have adopted a generic approach that regards caring as a role that, to some degree, transcends distinctions such as gender, age or client-group status. This is not to deny that such distinctions are of importance in structuring the experience of caring, and in the chapters that follow we explore their impact, but to assert that there is a sufficiently common core to caring to allow one to look across such groupings and see a shared set of experiences and problems. There are also ethical and policy reasons for treating carers as a category in their own right rather than, as commonly happens, subordinating them to the disability of the person for whom they care. The perception of caring as a generic activity has been reinforced by the activities of the carer lobby led by the Carers National Association, and the politics of caring have been much advanced by this perception. The generic approach has also been important in underwriting new service developments for informal carers, providing a focus for innovation and information, in which the work of the King's Fund Informal Carers Unit has been particularly important. Finally, looking across the client groups brings a number of advantages. Many of the problems faced by carers are common, and there are significant insights to be gained from exploring them as a unity. Important contrasts can also be revealed; the problems may be shared but the ways they are perceived and the forms of help that are offered, as we shall see, vary between service sectors.

The study on which this book draws looked at a range of carers:

- Older people with physical disabilities.
- Older people with mental health problems, mainly dementia.
- Younger adults with physical disabilities.
- Younger adults with mental health problems.
- Younger adults with learning disabilities.

The incorporation of mental health problems was unusual in a study of caring, and in Chapter 7 we explore the rationale for doing this and the analytic and policy benefits to be gained. Caring for an adult with learning disabilities is also sometimes seen as 'different', and we discuss the significance of these differences and the conflicts around them more fully in Chapter 6. The only significant group omitted were the carers of mentally or physically disabled children, reflecting what we felt were different normative expectations underlying the care of a child. A fuller account of the study and of the sample, which was obtained from surveys of the general population, is contained in the Appendix.

The concept of caring

The concept of caring is a mixed one, drawing on a number of elements. The first centres on the performance of tasks of a supportive character where these go beyond the normal reciprocities common between adults. Caring means doing things for people that they cannot do for themselves, and personal care tasks such as lifting, toileting and washing provide the clearest examples. It is often difficult, however, to distinguish between caring and the patterns of personal tending common within family and gender relations, with many women traditionally performing tasks for their spouses and families that would be classified as 'caring' if provided by men in reverse. Waerness (1984) draws a conceptual distinction between 'caring' and the 'servicing' work that women perform for husbands and children, distinguishing both from what she would see as genuinely reciprocal forms of support within a relationship.

Allied to the emphasis on caring tasks is the perception that caring involves physical labour, often hard physical labour. Much of the early exploratory work emphasized the daily grind of caring – the lifting, the cleaning, the feeding. This emphasis arose in part from a wish to de-romanticize caring, to take it away from a preoccupation with love and show how much of it was onerous work. The emphasis on physical tasks also arose from the early focus in the literature on carers of physically disabled, often older, people whose needs were of that nature; and for many researchers and practitioners, the performance of physical tasks has remained the defining feature of caring.

The second element in the meaning of caring is kinship obligation. Caring almost always takes place within a context of kinship (Evandrou *et al.* 1986; Finch 1989; Qureshi and Walker 1989). The support neighbours offer is typically limited, and they are rarely involved in intimate or physical care (Wenger 1984; Green 1988; Sinclair 1990; Hills 1991). Where friends or neighbours are closely involved it is usually because some earlier social experience has transformed these relationships into primary social bonds. In this book, we confine ourselves to 'primary' carers and we do not explore the 'informal sector' in the wider sense of community or neighbourhood support.

Third, caring is closely associated with emotion. Caring relations if not defined by love, are frequently associated with and energized by it, although in more complex and ambiguous ways than the normative picture might suggest. Roy Parker (1981) argued for the importance of distinguishing conceptually between 'caring about' and 'caring for' someone, and suggested that the term 'tending' should be substituted for the second. Although his argument has been widely acknowledged, the shift in terminology has not taken place. Graham (1983) argues that the two elements are intimately linked and that this linkage has special significance for the ways women, in particular, construct their caring role. Emotion is significant in a second way also. It is not just that love and other such feelings underwrite the bonds of obligation, contributing both to why people give care and to the experience of caring, but that caring represents a form of emotional labour in itself (Hochschild 1983; James 1989; Delphy and Leonard 1992). Carers do not simply do things for people, they can also support them with encouragement, personal attention and conversation that endorses their sense of identity and worth. Offering such support is part of the activity of caring.

Co-residence also forms a significant element in the construction of caring, though it is not a necessary part of it. Caring can take place between households and this is particularly characteristic where the cared-for person is an elderly parent (Green 1988). Co-residence is, however, as Qureshi and Walker demonstrate, highly influential in defining who within a family ends up as the carer, overriding factors such as gender and relationship (Qureshi and Walker 1989; Arber and Ginn 1991; Glendinning 1992). Sharing a household radically affects the experience of caring, and co-residence alerts us to the important ways in which caring is not just about the performance of tasks, but the *consequences of a relationship*. Carers' lives can be restricted because they share the limitations imposed on the life of the cared-for person, or because they share their homes with somebody whose behaviour disturbs daily life. The latter is particularly important for carers of people with dementia, or mental health problems or learning disabilities that result in behaviourial problems, where the consequences of sharing your life and household can be more significant in determining your experiences as a carer than any tasks performed.

Last, caring involves a feeling of *being responsible* for the cared-for person. This sense stems from the obligation that underpins these relationships: most carers feel that they are in some sense responsible for the situation of the person for whom they care. Carers commonly express a feeling that they represent 'the bottom line', or that they ultimately have to 'carry the can' for the person's support. This can mean monitoring the situation, negotiating with services, stepping up involvement as the need for it grows, adjusting actions to meet any service shortfall. In cases where the cared-for person has no need for physical help, the sense of 'being responsible' is the primary element in care-giving and, we would argue, represents the core feature that underlines all care-giving. Of course the assumption of responsibility is open to challenge. The disability critique in particular rejects the idea that someone other than the disabled person could be 'responsible' for his or her life. We shall return to this question later, only noting at this point that the sense of responsibility is fundamental to how carers experience their role and is reflected in the assumptions of service providers also.

Caring takes place in a relationship

This is a book about carers. They are the focus of our study, and in it we attempt to look at their needs and wishes, relating these to the assumptions and practices of service providers. In doing this, we incorporate into the analysis a concern for their interests *per se*, and we do not simply see their support in instrumental terms.

But caring takes place in a relationship. As important as the carer is the cared-for person. They, after all, are the reason why the caring exists, and it is the presence of their difficulties that transforms a family or social relationship into a caring one. The disability critique has rightly argued that caring cannot be examined separately from the needs and wishes of disabled people. Failing to address these directly creates dependence on others, creates 'caring'. Focusing exclusively on the carer is, moreover, demeaning to the disabled person, who is made into an adjunct of somebody else – no longer the subject of their own life.

There are public policy reasons also that limit the degree to which one can focus exclusively on the carer. 'Carers' are constituted as a subject by the relationship of obligation and care that they have with a disabled person. They feature in public policy by virtue of that relationship. They have always, therefore, to be seen in the context of it, and the perception of their needs can never wholly transcend that relationship.

By the same token, we would argue, it is not possible to focus exclusively on the disabled person, ignoring the existence of the carer and excluding them from moral concern (we are only addressing here situations where there is such a carer or family helper). Caring is embedded in relationships of obligation such as marriage, parenthood, kinship, in which people feel responsible for spouses, children or parents, and obliged to give care. These are not voluntary relationships, and these feelings of obligation have consequences for their lives – often, as we shall see, severe consequences. To ignore this fact and focus exclusively on the disabled person is unacceptable.

The element of obligation also affects how the carer's interest is treated within public policy. Carers are bound into relationships that mean they do not simply give up when the balance of interest turns against continuing. Carers carry on caring against their own interests. Simply to regard them in utilitarian fashion as subject to a form of rational calculation of costs and benefit in which they cease to give care once the former outweighs the latter is to miss that nature of the ties that bind them. And it is precisely because of these ties that public agencies have a moral, as opposed to a simply instrumental, relationship with them. Public agencies cannot treat carers as they might more distant members of the informal network such as neighbours, where there is an assumption that they will withdraw if the involvement becomes too burdensome. Carers pose moral responsibilities to welfare agencies precisely because they cannot be assumed to pursue their own interests in a straightforward way. For this reason their needs and interests must be incorporated into public policy. The models for doing so are the subject of the next chapter.

Chapter 2 CARERS IN THE SERVICE SYSTEM

In this chapter our focus turns from the carer to service provision, and we begin to explore the ways in which carers fit into the service system and the nature of service response to them. The chapter establishes some of the analytic categories that are employed later in the book. It divides into four sections. The first explores the ambiguous position of carers within the service system, outlining the four models of response adopted by agencies. The second discusses what counts as a 'service' for carers, developing the implications of this for the analysis of service provision, and describing the role of front-line service providers and exploring the process whereby carers are, or are not, incorporated into their practice. In the third section we discuss the nature of 'policy' in relation to carers, examining how it is constructed at the front line in the three service sectors. Last, we turn to the question of negotiation, suggesting that service receipt needs to be understood as the product of a process of negotiation between the service provider and the carer.

The ambiguous position of carers: four models

Carers occupy an ambiguous position in relation to service provision. They lie on the margins of the social care system: in one sense within its remit, part of its concerns and responses; in another, beyond its remit, part of the taken-for-granted reality against which welfare services operate. Carers exist off-centre to service provision. The relationship between the two is uncertain and ill-defined. Carers are not clients or patients, and they are rarely the direct focus of an intervention; and yet at the same time they are clearly part of the complexities of care that service providers have to recognize. As a result, agencies have difficulties in conceptualizing their relationship with carers; and this conceptual ambiguity extends to policymakers and researchers also. Much of the research in this field fails to come to grips with these problems, though they are central to questions of evaluation and the definition of outcomes.

We suggest that there are four models or ideal types of the response of service agencies to carers. In earlier work, Twigg (1989a) distinguished three models: carers as resources, as co-workers and as co-clients. We now add a fourth, that of the superseded carer. These models are not held exclusively, and agencies and service providers shift between the different frames of reference in response to the particularities of the situation.

Carers as resources

Carers as resources reflects the predominant reality of social care. The majority of help that comes to frail and disabled people does so from the informal sector. Care inputs from the informal sector vastly outweigh those from the formal (Walker 1982; Wicks 1982). There is little evidence to support the anxieties that have at times been expressed about the declining willingness or ability of families to support frail older people (Moroney 1976; Brody 1981; Wicks 1982; Parker 1990a), and this pattern of informal predominance is likely to continue (Finch 1989).

Informal care thus represents the 'given', the taken-for-granted social reality against which agencies operate. As a result, agencies regard carers as a form of resource, though a form of resource that is unlike other resources available to public agencies. It is, in general, free (both to the recipients of care and the agencies). For the latter it represents a classic free good. No cost – at least in this model – attaches to it. Its availability largely results from long-term social factors such as demography and family obligation and this means it is not subject to simple laws of supply and demand. Last, informal care has a normative priority over that of formal care. Within the mixed economy of welfare, some inputs have a prior status. There is an assumption among service providers and the wider public that informal care in some sense comes first; and there is a tendency to assume that the social care system need only step in when informal support is unavailable. Although this form of residualism – as we shall see when we turn to the other models – is not the only response of agencies to carers, it is a central feature of how they perceive carers, and it underpins the way in which carers are seen as part of the 'given' resources within the community. Informal care provides the backdrop to formal provision, but in doing so it exists prior to and quite separate from it.

What are the implications of this model for how carers are defined? Here the term 'carer' is employed very broadly, and carers are seen to include all potential informal supporters (see Table 1). At times the term becomes coterminous with the informal sector or the 'community' in general. All helpers are potentially co-opted by this approach, and no great distinction is made between the help given by friends, neighbours, distant kin, or closely involved carers. The resource model places its central focus on the cared-for person; and the carer only features as part of the background – albeit a vital resource background. Thus although agencies may be concerned to understand better the character of this background resource through research or other forms of increasing their knowledge, they are not primarily concerned with the interests of the carers themselves. Concern with carer welfare in this model is marginal or non-existent; and the potential conflict of interest between the carer and the cared-for person is ignored. The primary aim of intervention by the agency is the maintenance and perhaps marginal increase in levels of informal support; and

Table 1 Four models of carers

	Carers as resources	*Carers as co-workers*	*Carers as co-clients*	*Superseded carer*
Definition of carer	Very wide	Wide	Narrow	'Relatives'
Focus of interest	Disabled person	Disabled person with some instrumental recognition of the carer	Carer	Disabled person and carer, but separately
Conflict of interest	Ignored	Partly recognized	Recognized fully, but one way	Recognized, but in relation to both carer and disabled person
Aim	Care maximization and minimization of substitution	Highest quality of care for the disabled person. Well-being of carer as means to this	Well-being of the carer	Well-being of carer and independence for the disabled person, but seen as separate

concern will be expressed lest service support undermine or take over from what is seen as the prior family responsibility. Fear of the substitution of formal for informal support will predominate.

Carers as co-workers

The second model is of carers as co-workers. Here agencies aim to work alongside the informal sector, interweaving their support with that of the carers. Carers are seen as co-workers in a joint care enterprise, in which the traditional divisions between formal and informal care are transcended. In practice, such attempts often prove problematic, and Abrams and others have analysed the discordant assumptions that underlie the two systems (Froland 1981; Bulmer 1986; Abrams *et al.* 1989).

The definition of a carer in this model is wide. As with the resource approach, it encompasses all the potential sources of help in the community, friends and neighbours as well as kin, though with a slightly stronger emphasis on the primary carer. The main focus of the approach is still on the disabled person, but in a way that recognizes the instrumental importance of the morale of the carer, high carer morale contributing both to the likelihood that caregiving will continue to be offered and to the quality of that care. The co-worker model thus encompasses the carer's interest and well-being within its concerns, but on an essentially instrumental basis. The primary aim remains one of providing high-quality care for the cared-for person. Conflicts of interest in this model are partly recognized, but are usually submerged under an assumption that carers do primarily want to care and that assisting them to do so is the most important way for agencies to relate to carers.

Carers as co-clients

In this model, carers are regarded as clients, as people in need of help in their own right. Services are aimed at relieving their situation and enhancing their morale. The use of the term 'carer' is confined narrowly, applying only to those who are heavily involved in caring. Unlike the resource or co-worker models where agencies aim to incorporate as much of the informal sector as possible, here definitional boundaries are drawn tightly around the most highly stressed and heavily burdened. By this means the agency is able to limit the extent of its moral responsibility, confining it only to the most acute cases.

The focus of intervention is the carer and his or her needs, and his or her well-being is a valued outcome *per se*. This may in some cases be pursued at the expense of that of the cared-for person, at least in the short term. Institutional respite, with all the problems that that can entail (Hasselkus and Brown 1983; Wright 1986; Levin *et al.* 1989; Twigg *et al.* 1990a) offers the clearest example of such an emphasis. The conflict of interest between the carer and the cared-for person is fully recognized, though the emphasis is on the problems that this poses for the carer.

The superseded carer

Here the aim is not to support or underwrite the care-giving relationship, but to transcend or supersede it. There are two routes to this model. One starts from a concern with the disabled person and with maximizing their independence. The aim is to intervene in ways that result in their no longer having to rely on a carer. The aim is not to ease the lot of carers so much as to free disabled people from relationships of dependence. In some situations, particularly those of disabled adults being cared for by parents, the relationship may itself be seen as constricting to the disabled individual's personal growth. This model of response has been particularly influential in relation to people with learning disabilities, as well as for younger physically disabled adults and people diagnosed as schizophrenic. Its use in relation to carers of older people has been limited; these are not caring relationships that agencies have, by and large, been concerned to see superseded. The second route comes from a concern for the carer. Maximizing the independence of the disabled or older person will potentially dispense with the need for care, and with that, the burdens that fall on the carer. Sometimes it is also appropriate to think in terms of supporting a carer in the decision to give up caring. Taking the well-being of a carer seriously can involve accepting that only the cessation of caring will result in any significant improvement in morale, as the work of Levin and her colleagues demonstrated (Levin *et al.* 1989).

Carers on this superseded model tend not to be described as such. The word is replaced by terms like 'relatives' or 'family' that are more neutral and do not imply the same levels of obligations and responsibility that are suggested by the term 'carer'. The focus of the intervention is on either the disabled person or the carer, depending on which route has been the influential one. Either way, the carer and the disabled person are seen as separate beings. The conflict of interest is fully recognized, and from the viewpoint of both individuals. The valued outcome of intervention is independence for both the carer and the disabled person.

The four models outlined above represent ideal types of response. Agencies do not draw exclusively on any one in framing their response to carers. The emphasis placed, however, does vary systematically. We have noted this particularly in relation to different client groups, though there is evidence also that different models are stressed at different levels of the organization. Front-line workers, particularly those with social work training, tend to be drawn to the co-worker model, whereas managerial staff tend to see things more in terms of the resource model, though sometimes combined with an instrumental emphasis on carers as the most cost-effective means of supporting disabled people. There are also differences in emphasis between socially- and medically-oriented practitioners, with a greater tendency for medical staff to regard carers simply as an unquestioned background resource than is the case with social care professionals who tend to be more aware of carers as co-clients. We shall explore these differences in the following chapters.

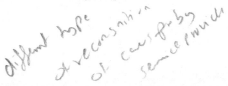

What counts as a service for carers?

What counts as a service for carers is by no means a straightforward matter. As we have seen, carers are rarely the direct focus of an intervention. They are not – primarily – clients, but feature within the service system by virtue of their relationship with a client. They are not catered for by one particular service, but are pervasive through the service system: where clients are, there also are carers – in potential at least.

It is helpful when thinking about services for carers to see them as existing through a series of levels (Figure 1), starting from the small-scale and specific and moving to the pervasive and general. Two dimensions define this movement. The first is the degree to which the services operate specifically with carers in mind – in other words, the degree of incorporation of the carer's interest (we shall return to the question of incorporation more fully below). The second is the scope of the scheme: ranging from small-scale, specific services, through mainstream services, to the global level of the service system as a whole.

At the simplest level we have services that are unambiguously provided in order to support a carer. They ofter have the word carer or relative in their title. Carer support groups or Crossroads Care Attendants provide classic examples.

Figure 1 Services for carers

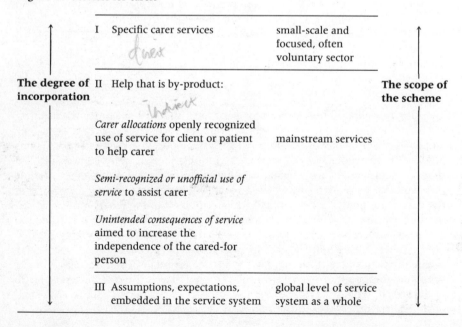

↑	I Specific carer services	small-scale and focused, often voluntary sector	↑
The degree of incorporation	II Help that is by-product: *Carer allocations* openly recognized use of service for client or patient to help carer *Semi-recognized or unofficial use of service* to assist carer *Unintended consequences of service* aimed to increase the independence of the cared-for person	mainstream services	**The scope of the scheme**
↓	III Assumptions, expectations, embedded in the service system	global level of service system as a whole	↓

Such services tend to be small in scale, and they are often either innovations or located in the voluntary sector. It is these services that have traditionally been regarded as central to the support of carers.

At the next level, we have support that comes to the carer as a by-product of services aimed at the cared-for person. Carers are helped by services that are not primarily aimed at them but at the cared-for person. Sometimes this happens in an overt way, as for example when a place is provided in a day hospital for the cared-for person but with the intention of relieving the carer. Sometimes the intention is more mixed, as for example with day care for people with learning disabilities where the primary purpose is educational, but where it is recognized that the placement also helps the parents. These are not so much carer 'services', as carer allocations. Carers are also helped as a by-product of mainstream services where these operate to increase the independence of the cared-for person. Here the focus is straightforwardly on the cared-for person, but the knock-on effects for the carer can be considerable. It was clear from the carer interviews that form the basis of this study that it was mainstream services organized primarily around the cared-for person that provided the bulk of support to carers.

Last, there are global service assumptions and practices. These form the context within which the first two levels are contained. Service providers make assumptions about carers – their availability, their duties, their likely involvement – and to some degree structure their provision in the light of those. These embedded assumptions and practices can have major implications for carers through their impact on, for example, the way the ambulance service is organized, or the assumptions that hospital consultants make about the availability of spouses to care. They are not carer 'services', but represent the impact the system as a whole has upon the lives of carers. Exploration of the role of services in relation of carers needs to be extended from its current remit to encompass this third level, and to examine the network of embedded assumptions, rules and practices that structure the service system.

We now turn to the implications of this understanding of what constitutes a service for carers for the approach taken in this book. First, the study is not confined to a specific service, but ranges across the service system as a whole. Most evaluative work on services for carers has focused on particular interventions or schemes. Work in this vein has been valuable, but it misses much of the experience of service receipt, which is complex, fragmented and interactive. Simply to focus on one intervention is to miss that reality. As Hills points out, carers have a range of needs and the effectiveness of one service may depend on the availability of another: 'a sitting service without the information service that referred the carer or the support group that enabled the carer to cope with the guilt engendered by using the service may [make] little difference'(Hills 1991: 78). In this study we look at services in a complex way, taking on board the implications of all three of the levels identified above.

The second implication concerns the limitations of a 'units of service' approach. By this we mean the tradition of service analysis that focuses on the evaluation of the impact of defined units of service. The approach is embedded in the quantitative tradition, particularly that which attempts to cost inputs. Discrete units of service are, however, an inadequate way in which to conceptualize how carers receive (or do not receive) support from the service system. If we take the example of the third level described above, it is less a question of discrete units of service, than of the network of assumptions and practices concerning caring that are embedded in service provision generally. It is not so much that the ambulance or the hospital consultant represent a 'service' for the carer as that their practice can have a significant impact on the situation of the carer, for better or worse. A units of service approach is overly narrow and cannot capture these wider aspects that are so significant in relation to carers. Pulling back from such an approach furthermore allows us to avoid the artificial separation of inputs and process. It is central to the experience of carers that the ways in which things are done is part of what is done. Presenting a more fluid, deconstructed account that ranges across the service system as a whole and addresses *how* as well as *what* allows us to reflect these complexities.

Embarking on such a process of deconstruction also allows us to reflect the significance of the distinction made above between carer 'services' and carer 'allocations'. It is clear, returning to the second level, that as important as the existence of a unit of service, like a day-care place, is the question of whether it is used in order to support a carer. It is this decision by the service provider that determines whether or not a 'service' exists for the carer. Services of this type have an inevitably fluid and discretionary quality to them; their very existence is rooted in the individual allocative decisions of service providers. They are 'created' out of existing resources. The existence of a service for a carer is thus not straightforward or fixed, but rests upon discretion, interpretation and use. For this reason it is not always possible to say definitively what provision exists for carers in an area, since it is the actual use of resources that is the critical feature. What is significant, therefore, and what we address in this book, is not specific carer services or units of service, but the way in which carers relate to the service system as a whole.

Deconstructing the service system

In the research study that underpins this book, we adopted a methodology that involved starting from the viewpoint of the individual carer and analysing where, how and whether they got help with the difficulties that faced them. Unlike other studies our sample was not recruited through service providers, but from a natural population (see Appendix). We were thus able to track from the carers to the service providers rather than vice versa as is more commonly the case. In doing so we did not pre-empt what services were relevant or whether help was in fact received, but allowed carers to lead us to what were the significant sources of support. This enabled us to see service support in a deconstructed way, as a series of possibilities, of contingent comings together of help, rather than as a coherent and unitary system. This approach finds echoes in the recent changes in community care, part of whose aim has been to break up the service monoliths, replacing them by a more flexible response that transcends the 'irrationalities' and perverse incentives of the current, service-based, system. In a similar way our analysis attempts to break up the rigidities of a units-of-service approach and replace it with a more fluid picture of interaction and involvement, in which non-receipt and absence of response are also important.

In order to pursue this deconstruction we focus on two aspects: (1) the front line of service interaction and (2) what service providers actually do for carers. Taking the latter first, it is clear that service providers do – or potentially do – a variety of things for carers. They offer direct practical help of a hands-on variety. This can be in the form of substituting for the carer in order to lighten their load, as for example with a district nurse giving a bath; or in order to create space for the carer to relax as, for example, through the help of a sitter. Service providers also provide indirect help when they take decisions relating to the cared-for person, but in the light of what they know concerning the carer – for example, where the hospital consultant delays a discharge in order to help the carer. Service providers are also of central importance to carers by virtue of their role as linking agents, referring carers to other service providers or forms of help. This aspect of their work is commonly analysed under the simple term 'referral', and covers the range of activities whereby service providers relate their practice to other forms of help. We distinguish four forms. The first is *allocation* where the service provider has direct command over the provision of a resource. An example of this would be the direct allocation by the psychiatrist of a place at the day hospital. The second is *strong referral.* This is where a practitioner assesses and refers to another service and where there is the strong expectation that the referral will be acted upon. An example of this would be a social worker referring a client to day care but where the client may have to wait until a place becomes available and where the social workers will not themselves determine between different candidates. Here the assessment of eligibility and the actual provision, though linked, are separated. Strong referrals are only made by certain service providers, such as GPs and social workers, who are relatively powerful and who operate on a professional model. Such referrals are nearly always made within the service provider's service sector: necessarily so, since the separate assessments and allocations are still linked, and it is impossible to achieve this across service sectors, and sometimes even across services. *Weak referrals* are where the service provider passes on a referral to another service with the expectation that the service will assess and possibly allocate. An example of this would be where a GP makes a referral to the home help service or to a social worker. (The GP may not always understand it as such, confusion in expectations as to whether it is a weak or a strong referral is a fruitful source of conflict between service providers.) Last, there are *recommendations* where the service provider suggests a source of help to the client or carer but leaves it up to them to apply.

Service providers are also involved in a broad set of activities concerned with giving the carer emotional support and the opportunity to talk about the situation. For some practitioners, such as social workers, this may take place within a conscious framework such as psychotherapeutic counselling or the 'ventilation' of feeling. Other service providers, like home helps, are also involved in these activities though at a less self-conscious level. Service providers are also involved in talk of a more directive type. Psychoeducation for the parents of someone diagnosed as schizophrenic is a specific example of this. Advice on where to get help or how to manage difficulties is a more general one.

Mapping the service system: the focus on the front line

It is clear as we run through this list of activities that not only do they represent a range of tasks in the support of carers, but also of roles and positions within the network of community care. The service providers involved include such diverse personnel as home-help organizers, psychiatrists, social workers, GPs, hospital consultants, managers of voluntary-sector day centres, key workers in a mental handicap team and occupational therapists. These personnel exhibit considerable differences of status and power. They also vary greatly in the levels of discretion they exercise, the use of discretion varying with the degree to which they draw on a professional model of practice. Some of these service providers, like social workers, operate within line-management systems in which they are to some degree expected to carry out organizational policy; others, like GPs, are relatively independent agents.

There are difficulties in presenting a coherent account of community care as it relates to carers when the individuals operating it are so diverse in their roles and organizational positions. There is little work that has attempted to look across the care system in this way. Hunter and his colleagues' study of provision for elderly people was a notable exception, though it did not present a framework for analysing the different tasks, roles and statuses that are involved (Hunter *et al.* 1988). The most fruitful approach for the analysis of this service territory has been that of Lipsky in his *Street Level Bureaucracy* (1980).

Street level bureaucracy

Lipsky's analysis is concerned with front-line workers in public service organizations. His street level bureaucrats include many of the service providers that are of relevance to carers: GPs, social workers, home-care organizers. Street level bureaucrats interact directly with citizens and exercise discretion over aspects of their lives. They work in situations where resources are chronically inadequate; where demand is greater than supply; where the goals of agencies are vague and conflicting; and where it is difficult to define performance or measure the achievement of goals. The central feature of their work is the exercise of discretion. This, however, is not total. Street level bureaucrats work within a context of rules and directives that are shaped by the policy élite. To the extent that they are professionals, the exercise of discretion will be openly acknowledged and legitimate. But discretion is also exercised by staff who are not professionals, and who often occupy quite lowly positions. Lipsky outlines three reasons why discretion is intrinsic to these jobs. First, many of the situations faced by these workers are too complex to reduce to what Lipsky terms 'programatic formats'. Second, they typically require responses to a human dimension of the situation, and require sensitive personal handling. Third, the exercise of discretion in these cases encourages the citizen to believe that the worker is indeed focused on their well-being, and this underwrites the legitimation of welfare services.

Lipsky's analysis is cast at the level of the 'dilemmas' human public service of workers, and it is a limitation of the work that it does not engage fully with more structural and functional aspects. To these three reasons, we would therefore add a fourth, that concerning 'transparency', or rather the avoidance of it. By transparency we mean the ability of an organization to make its allocative principles explicit, rational and public. Welfare systems, embedded as they are in local and national politics, have traditionally avoided such transparency. Relying on the discretion of street level bureaucrats allows the organization to fragment and obscure its decisions, and this is central to the ways in which such services have traditionally been rationed. We shall return to this in Chapter 11.

Closely linked to the exercise of discretion is the fact of limited resources. Street level bureaucrats work where the resource problems are endemic and ultimately irresolvable. The better the service, the more responsive to needs, the greater the demand. Demand in these areas is itself interactive. As Lipsky states: 'It is a function not only of the expressions of clients but also of the willingness of government to offer services and to record or acknowledge client responses.' Demand is something that organizations can control and create by such techniques such as structuring the material and social context of service interactions and teaching the client the proper expectations to hold.

Lipsky's analysis has obvious applications to the circumstances of carers. The three aspects of discretion, uncertain policy aims and resource constraint are central, and together provide the framework within which service provision for carers must be understood. Services in relation to carers are controlled by service providers who exercise discretion; and the ambiguous and uncertain position of carers *vis-à-vis* the service system reinforces this element. Policy aims for carers are vague and ill-defined; we shall explore this further below. Last, carers relate to a field where resource constraint is central; this point is such an inescapable part of the reality of service provision in this area that we will digress briefly to emphasize it.

Resource constraint

Social care agencies operate in a context where budgets are limited (fixed by the political process) and where demand does not directly affect the level of supply. This contrasts with welfare systems that rest, for example, on insurance principles and where demand to some extent affects supply. Although the concept of 'assessment for need' is widely current within professional and policy rhetoric, the reality is that services are rationed, and that allocation is always made in the context of resource constraint. In practice there is no pure assessment of need separate from judgements about availability. These are also service sectors where there is a chronic shortage of resources. The quantification of this is a matter of contention, and cannot be divorced from judgements that are by their nature political. However, there is a consensus in the field that the social care system, if not underresourced, is under continuing resource pressure. The dominant experience within health and social services is one of lack of resources. Within these service sectors, support for carers is a particularly poorly resourced area, with the result that carers experience a double pressure – operating within a low-budget area of a constrained service sector.

As a result, carers typically receive very little help and, as we shall see, there are major discrepancies between what service providers regard as legitimate aspirations in regard to support for carers and what they are actually able to deliver. To this degree, what Davies terms the 'horizontal target efficiency' (defined as the degree to which individuals in the target category receive the intervention) is so poor that 'vertical target efficiency' (defined as the degree to which individuals who receive the intervention fall within the target category) is almost total (Davies and Challis 1986). As a result no one in the study received a service that could have been regarded as 'inappropriate'. Some received more than others and we shall explore why in greater detail below. But none received services that could be regarded as unnecessary or excessive.

Incorporating carers

The resource constraints reinforce the exercise of discretion, since social care agencies typically ration support in ways that are covert. Rationing is performed by front-line workers who have to make decisions balancing needs and resources in individual cases. In doing so they have to decide how and in what ways carers will be incorporated into their practice. Incorporation is, however, only the last stage of a complex process whereby carers come to interact with service provision. This process can be analysed in terms of three stages: coming into the orbit of the service, visibility and incorporation.

The first stage is that of *coming into the orbit* of the service. This can happen in a variety of ways. It can occur as a result of certain events such as the hospitalization of the cared-for person, since it is often only as a consequence of a fall or other medical crisis that the carer and the cared-for person comes into the orbit of services. It can also occur as a result of the carer him or herself seeking help, calling at the town hall or going to the GP. It can also result from a structured outreach by the service, for example where an attempt is made to contact and place on a register all people in the locality with learning disabilities. However it occurs, what matters is that the carer has come into the orbit of services.

The next stage is one of *becoming visible*. This applies both literally and metaphorically. Some carers remain literally invisible to service providers because they never meet them, they never call at the house or look beyond their consulting room. Others remain so metaphorically because the service provider fails to perceive their involvement or does not recognize them as carers. Some of the barriers to visibility relate to the contexts in which service providers practice, others to their professional ideology and work cultures: whichever is the case, how carers are perceived is central to their experience of service provision.

Finally, there is the stage of *incorporation*. How far and in what ways the carer is incorporated into the practice of the service provider will depend to some degree on which of the four models of the appropriate relationship between carers and service provision predominates. There are clear differences, for example, between a carer who is incorporated as a co-client and one who is incorporated as a co-worker. Carers as resources are only incorporated in an implicit way as part of the background to the service provider's practice. The superseded carer is, of course, incorporated only in the very restricted sense of being consciously excluded. How the carer is incorporated will affect the interactions that occur between the carer and the service provider, and the decisions that are made. It will determine how far and in what ways the carer's interest is taken into account. Incorporation is thus a wider concept than simply allocation. It encompasses a range of responses, and may not involve allocation at all. In the chapters that follow we will analyse the ways in which various service providers incorporate carers into their practice, exploring the factors that determine whether they become visible and the paths that lead them into the orbit of services.

What is the nature of 'policy' for carers?

Service providers at the front line operate within a policy context, and we now turn to the question of what constitutes policy for carers. There has been a long-running debate in the public administration literature concerning the nature of policy and its role within organizations (Smith and May 1980; Barrett and Fudge 1981; Webb and Wistow 1982; Ham and Hill 1984; Hunter *et al.* 1988). The protagonists divide broadly into the *rationalist/managerialist* view and the *behaviourial/pluralist* critique. The former is a top-down approach that assumes that organizations – in this case welfare agencies – are goal-directed, and that they exist in order to give expression to policies that are set at the top of the organization. It is an approach that embodies what Elmore (1981) terms 'forward mapping' in the sense of an account that starts from stated objectives and pursues the logic of their implementation down through the organization. Policy and implementation are regarded as separate. The task of the manager is to ensure the detailed implementation of policy; and running organizations is regarded as a constant struggle to obtain control over implementation. It is a rationalistic account, and it contains strongly normative elements. Smith and May (1980) argue that it represents an ideal of policy making rather than an account of its realities.

The behaviourial/pluralist tradition presents a critique of this view. It questions how far government or other agencies do in fact identify clear policies, arguing instead that policies are by their nature vague and complex. They are rarely couched in specific terms, and they can embody a series of conflicting values and aims. Sometimes they are deliberately obscure, and that obscurity is at the heart of their political character. Ham and Hill (1984) indeed suggest that it is dangerous to assume that there is a recognizable entity called 'policy'; and they argue that it is 'difficult to treat it as a very specific or concrete phenomenon' (Ham and Hill 1984: 11).

The behaviourial/pluralist view is a 'backward mapping', bottom-up approach. It questions the assumption that policymakers exercise a determining influence over what happens. Rather than starting from the expression of policy intent, it focuses on the specific behaviours that take place at the front line of the organization. As Wildavsky (1979: 387) argues: 'policy is a process as well as a product'. Though the approach regards the policymaker's perspective as important, it does not assume that this is the only influence on front-line actors. Policy and implementation are not separated; policy is seen as created through the process of implementation. Policy does not exist primarily in formal policy statements, but is embodied in the actions of front-line workers. It is 'revealed only in the content and style of a decision or stream of decisions' (Webb and Wistow 1982: 12). The approach is echoed by Lipsky (1980: xii, original emphasis): 'the decisions of street level bureaucrats, the routines they establish and the devices they invent to cope with uncertainties and work pressures, effectively *become* the public policies they carry out'.

In this study we have adopted a concept of 'policy' that is broadly within the behaviourial/pluralist tradition. This is partly because we believe that the approach is a superior one, certainly one that is better able to capture the realities of organizations, but also because it has affinities with our subject of study. The behaviourial/pluralist approach accepts that policy may be vague and contradictory, and that it is created at all levels of the organization. The approach is particularly apposite to a study of carers, where until recently few policy statements have been made, and those mostly of a very general nature. The issue in relation to carers is not one of a struggle for implementation, but of the actual forging of policy at the different levels of the organization. Carers have until recently existed in a policy vacuum. As a result nearly all the 'policy' that there is in relation to them is implicit, embedded in the everyday patterns of practice. This is what is effectively delivered by the organization, and that is what we shall examine in the chapters that follow. Although we conceive of 'policy' in this inclusive way it is important to retain certain distinctions, and we will explore the significance of these in relation to the three front-line service sectors.

The social services department

If we look at the nature of policy for carers within social service departments, there are three main ways in which it is embodied.

Explicit policy

The first represents policy in the classic sense of *explicit policy*, formally defined and determined at the top of the organization. In the case of social services, this is set by chief officers and senior managers with the involvement, to varying degrees, of councillors, and with the policy context in which they operate in turn influenced by government legislation and guidance. Policy in social services typically takes the form of reports to the social services committee, subsequently ratified in policy directives. Such overt policymaking in regard to carers has until recently been rare. Even now it is unusual for carers to be the subject of strategic policy documents, though they are increasingly mentioned in those relating to other groups. Part of this neglect has been as a result of the client groups to which carers relate. The client group that dominates policymaking in social services is children. This has always been the case and the combined effect of the legislative bias, which means that the majority of statutory obligations refer to children, and the impact of recurring scandals, have helped maintain this imbalance. As a result the care of elderly people, people with mental health problems, young physically disabled people and those with learning disabilities have had a lower priority in terms of formal policymaking. Carers predominantly relate to these client groups, and they thus share in that neglect.

A larger part of the absence of explicit policy for carers relates, however, to the ambiguous position they occupy in relation to social care agencies that we noted earlier. Social services had difficulty conceptualizing their relationship with carers, and this has resulted in a relative lack of overt policymaking for this group. It is also the case that until recently agencies were not under any pressure to develop such policy. The impact of the growing politicization of the issue which we noted in Chapter 1, and the moves within social services towards explicit objective-setting, exemplified in mission statements and community care plans, has, however, resulted in more formal policymaking for carers. The purchaser/provider split is likely to reinforce the trend towards policy definition.

Guidelines and regulations

Below the level of explicit policy is a network of *guidelines and regulations* governing the work of front-line practitioners. These are sometimes gathered together in practice guides, but more often exist in the form of memoranda or instructions from managers. They define, for example, what tasks the home help should or should not undertake; or they outline certain procedures that must be gone through before someone is admitted to a residential home. These regulations often relate to past scandals or problems. They are frequently defensive in tone, and often expressed in terms of what must *not* be done. Some are more strategic in aim, but this is usually where their intention is to ensure due consideration of the use of an expensive resource such as a place in a residential home. It is important to appreciate that their coverage is uneven. They are patchy and cannot be said of themselves to constitute a policy: they need to be read against the everyday patterns of service delivery. Once again carers rarely feature among these regulations, and in the past have done so largely in negative terms; thus it was common for home-help services to have a rule forbidding the allocation of the service to an elderly person who had a relative living locally. More recently at this level there have been moves in some authorities towards explicit guidelines requiring that the carer's perspective be included as part of the assessment.

Operative/implicit policy

Below the guidelines and regulations we have front-line practitioners. This is the level of *operative* or *implicit policy*. It is here that the most significant decisions in relation to carers are made; and it is here that we will place the main emphasis of our analysis. How implicit policy is constructed varies between the different service providers, and we describe this in greater detail in Chapters 4 to 6. It is useful at this stage, however, to distinguish three recurring sources (in addition to that of the formal policy of the organization).

Professional values The first is *professional values*. Not all practitioners in this field are professionals in the classic sense, and many like social workers are more commonly termed 'quasi-professionals'. They vary in the degree to which they draw upon an articulate body of knowledge as the basis for their practice. All however, through training and socialization in professional roles, internalize models of good practice, and these are important in guiding their actions and structuring the accounts they give of them.

Culture of the office The second major source of implicit policy is what we term the *culture of the office*. This operates most strongly in relation to service providers who have little or no formal training. The culture of the office represents the shared assumptions and understandings that service providers develop over time in conjunction with their colleagues. It includes general understandings about the nature of the job, and how it should be undertaken, as well as injunctions concerning how to deal with particular types of case, in the form of routinized responses. This embedded tradition of response arises most strongly where there are few explicit directives as to how the work should be done and where practitioners, sharing the same office, draw on one another in order to resolve their uncertainties collectively. The impact of the culture of the office is most powerful where practitioners have little in the way of professional training on which to draw and where there are few explicit directives as to how the work should be done.

Assumptive worlds Third, there are the personal values and attitudes of service providers. We term these *assumptive worlds*, meaning by this the network of assumptions and meanings that service providers bring to their work by virtue of their existence as social beings. In using assumptive worlds in this sense, we are defining its meaning more narrowly than has been the case in some work where it has been used to encompass all sources of interpretation and meaning. Here, however, we use it to denote the sources of meaning that derive from outside the working environment. Assumptive worlds are particularly important in relation to carers because the issues which they raise are rooted in ordinary-life assumptions concerning such matters as family, kinship obligation and gender relations. These assumptions will vary systematically between individuals according to factors such as social class. Their influence in forming implicit policy should not be underestimated. When practitioners work with children or marital problems they bring to their practice bodies of theory that structure their responses to these aspects of family life. In relation to care-giving, there is no equivalent body of theory; and as a result practitioners draw much more heavily on their personal experiences and values, although often in an implicit and unconscious way. As we shall see, assumptive worlds play a more significant role in the accounts of service providers who are untrained. Professional education appears in some degree to displace them – at least at the level of discourse. Whether it does so in substance is less clear, and it is important not to assume that the rationalistic accounts given by professionals of the bases of their practice represent complete ones.

The health service

Turning now to the health service, it is clear that 'policy' is constructed here in a different organizational context from that of social services. The major distinction lies in the role of the medical profession and the clinical autonomy of doctors. Doctors operate according to individual conceptions of clinical practice, and this means that the organization – here the health authority – has limited legitimate or actual control over their actions. The autonomy of doctors is, of course, subject to constraint, notably in the case of hospital doctors through the ability of the health authority to allocate resources to different areas of clinical practice. It remains the case, however, that these practitioners do not operate within a line management structure; and one cannot, therefore, describe their work in terms of the transmission of the formal policy of the organization. In relation to GPs, the autonomy is even greater since professional freedom is underwritten by their status as independent contractors. The growth of budget-holding strengthens this autonomy further. This is not to say that health authorities play no role in policymaking. Clearly they make strategic decisions about resources, and this role in determining priorities will increase with the purchaser/provider split. They also make policy statements, although in the past these have tended to relate to more peripheral areas of activity, with the major clinical sectors remaining under the control of doctors. In general, health authorities have found it easier to set policy in areas where professional interest and dominance are low, and they have also been more active in policymaking where the staff subject to the policy are non-medical.

Until recently, health authorities paid little attention to the issue of informal care. By and large they did not regard it as *their* issue, and the traditional preoccupation with the acute sector reinforced the disinclination to become involved. The situation is, however, changing, and there are signs, at least at the level of some regional health authorities, that the issue is beginning to be perceived as a health service one. Hospital discharge is likely to be a focus of tension in the new structures for health care, with pressure building up on trusts and acute units to discharge patients. Carers are pivotal figures in this process, and it is likely as a result that health authorities will develop a sharper and more instrumental interest in policymaking for this group.

Below the level of formal policy is the implicit policy of front-line workers, constructed in a similar way as in social services. Professional training and values are particularly significant in the health sector, and we shall discuss the role of these in relation to GPs and community nurses in the chapters that follow. The culture of the office has less relevance. It clearly does not apply to GPs whose practice is highly individualistic. It has some relevance to community nurses, though their contact with colleagues is limited; and the shared assumptions of the service, reinforced by nursing managers, is a better way to conceptualize their situation.

Last, assumptive worlds once again play a central role. How these different sources of implicit policy are woven together by the individual service providers is described in Chapter 5.

The voluntary sector

Policy in relation to the voluntary sector is a less easy concept to locate. 'Voluntary sector' is itself a notoriously unsatisfactory term with which to describe the variety of organizations, schemes and activities that are covered by this label, and Leat has discussed some of the problems of conceptualizing this area (Leat 1990). For our purposes the major distinction is between voluntary sector agencies that operate as quasi-service providers and those whose activities are more clearly in the campaigning/self-help/fund-raising modes. In relation to the latter group, it is problematic to speak of policy. Individuals in, for example, a self-help group may have *views* about the situation of carers, and the group may thus have an implicit stance, but it is not sensible to describe this as *policy*, at least on a direct parallel with that of formal agencies. In relation to the first group, however – those providing services – it is possible to talk about policy. Thus the voluntary sector day centre for people with Alzheimer's disease has a policy in relation to allocation. This is often implicit, operated informally through the priorities of the manager, though it may be closely tailored to the policies of the statutory agencies if these are providing funding.

The sources of implicit policy in this sector are once again diverse. National organizations like Age Concern or the National Schizophrenia Fellowship operate as policymakers, but their role at the level of the front-line worker is limited. Local groups retain considerable autonomy, and the motivations of individuals giving their time voluntarily mean that they are often unwilling to be subject to policy guidance or regulation (Thornton 1989, 1991). Some individuals in this sector are, of course, employed. Here there are closer parallels with the formal sector, although the articulation of policy remains weak. The culture of the office, the ideas shared among volunteers and workers as to what the enterprise is about, are of greater significance. Assumptive worlds, once again, play a major role.

Negotiation

This brings us to our final subject: that of the negotiation of services. So far in this chapter we have concentrated on the relationship between carers and service provision from the perspective of the service providers, discussing how agencies perceive their relationship with carers, the processes by which service providers do and do not incorporate carers into their practice and the ways in which implicit policy is constructed at this front line. It is important to recognize, however, that service provision is a two-way affair involving both the service provider and the user/carer. (Our primary focus in this study is on the carer, but the points we make apply as much to users.) Services are not allocated but negotiated. This truth contrasts in some degree with the dominant tradition of analysis in the field which is one that focuses on the rationality of allocation and in which decision-making about services is presented as wholly in the hands of service providers, judgements then being made as to the degree that pattern of allocation meets the policy aims of the agency. It is an approach that tends to conceive of service response rather narrowly in terms of the allocation of units of service; and we have already noted the limitation of this in relation to what constitutes 'services' for carers. Above all, it is an agency-dominated perspective in which service providers respond to certain objectively-given situations; and it ignores the degree to which users and carers themselves play a significant part in the negotiation of services.

We suggest instead that there is a realm of negotiation that lies between carers and service provision, and that carers themselves contribute to any response that is made or 'decision' that is reached. The definition of the situation, the conceptualization of need, the acceptability of the service that is offered – all are subject to a process of negotiation between the service provider and the carer to which the carer brings his or her perceptions and views. How carers interpret their situation, what they expect and think it legitimate to accept help with, how they judge its usefulness are all relevant to the process of negotiating services.

In arguing that service provision is a result of negotiation, we do not of course want to suggest that the parties to this are equal. Service provision takes place in a context of power in which service providers not only have control over the allocations but also to some degree over the definitions of the situation – of the nature and source of the problems or troubles (Gubrium 1989) that carers experience. In this process, certain sorts of discourse – particularly that of high status professionals operating with rationalistic frames of reference – are ascribed greater authority (Atkin 1991). Carers develop their views and expectations of services in the context of their contacts with service providers. Part of the power of practitioners lies in their capacity to teach appropriate expectations and responses to clients and patients (Sarri and Hasenfeld 1978; Lipsky 1980).

Much of the established literature about the capacity of service providers to control the definitions and teach clients appropriate roles has been concerned with the ways in which public service agencies develop techniques to manage and reduce demand. This is important: service providers do sometimes use their position *vis-à-vis* carers to limit requests for help or to embed people more firmly in their familial obligations. But it is not the whole story. As we shall see, service providers sometimes work to encourage carers to accept help, and this process of negotiating the service can be important in relation to services like respite that many carers are reluctant to accept. Service providers are sometimes also significant in encouraging people to perceive themselves as carers – as we shall see, an important stage for some individuals – to develop wider aspects of their lives and, even, to consider the possibility of giving up care.

The process of negotiation applies to all service delivery, but it is particularly significant in relation to carers. Why is this so? First, there is little in the way of an established tradition about appropriate support for carers. What *is* it legitimate to expect help with? What is too much, or too stressful? Should you as a carer be expected to bath your father-in-law, to help with the manual evacuation of bowels, or give up your job to care? These uncertainties apply also to the situation of older or disabled people contemplating help, but to a lesser degree. There is some tradition about the kinds of support that are available and legitimate. The role of the home help, for example, is widely understood and endorsed by older people. What is available and appropriate for carers is much less clear. There is a parallel lack of clarity on the part of service providers. As we have noted formal policy in relation to carers is even less defined than it is in relation to older people. Responding to the needs of carers is a relatively new injunction for service providers, who cannot therefore draw on an established service tradition.

Second, the situation in relation to carers is itself more subjective and open to interpretation and negotiation than is the case with, for example, disability which has a more directly concrete quality. We are, of course, aware that 'disability' is also a negotiated reality, but it is one to which certain benchmarks of an 'objective' nature can be applied and this is commonly done in the field as part of an attempt to focus the assessment process through the use of, for example, EDL (every day living) measures or mobility criteria. Caring does not fit well into this approach. To a limited degree one can apply such criteria, for example, the ability of the carer to lift the cared-for person. But as soon as one moves on to questions like does the carer *want* to give a bath, or does he or she want help in order to go out to work, one is into more fluid, subjective areas in which expectations, interpretation and volition are central. With the aspect of volition comes the possibility of persuasion and of manipulation – and on both sides. The process is an interactive one. Carers may adjust their behaviour and willingness in the light of their perception of what is or may become available. Their responses are not fixed but negotiable, and this applies to service providers as well. Volition is central to the situation and differs in degree from questions like, can you walk to the door or not. It affects the definition of 'need', and is a central aspect underwriting negotiation.

Chapter 3 *THE CARERS' EXPERIENCE*

Chapter 2 set the conceptual framework and policy context within which support for carers will be discussed. We now turn to the more detailed examination of the experiences and problems of carers, drawing directly on the study interviews. We concentrate in this chapter on the situation of carers of younger physically disabled adults and of older people with physical disabilities or mental frailty. These form what can be regarded as the paradigm case of caring in terms of which most of the literature and debate has been structured. Caring for younger adults with learning disabilities or mental health problems poses a slightly different set of problems, though as suggested in Chapter 1, ones that are still usefully seen within a common category of 'caring'. The differences and similarities, together with the responses of service providers, will be discussed in Chapters 7 and 8 which deal specifically with the carers of people with learning disabilities and mental health problems.

We now turn to the problems that carers experience, looking at what they do for the cared-for person and the sources of help that they draw upon.

Physical tending

Physical tending is sometimes regarded as the defining feature of informal care, and the literature has emphasized the hard physical labour that can be involved in caring and its impact on the carer's life and health (Glendinning 1983, 1985; Jones and Vetter 1984). Other studies have described in detail the physical tending commonly performed by carers (Bradshaw 1980; Nissel and Bonnerjea 1982; Glendinning 1983; Wright 1986; Lewis and Meredith 1988; Parker 1993), and the tasks undertaken by carers in this study were similar. The cared-for person needed help with bathing, dressing, getting in and out of bed, lifting, toileting, walking, taking medication and household activities. The amount and nature of physical care required varied with the disability. It can, however, be divided into four broad categories: personal care; the management of incontinence; medical and nursing care; and household tasks.

Personal care

Two features of personal care have an important bearing on the difficulties experienced by carers. The first is its intimate nature. Personal care involves touching, nakedness and contact with excreta and Ungerson has argued that it involves aspects of taboo that can pose problems in caring relationships (Ungerson 1983, 1987). The meaning of personal care is mediated by relationship and gender. Different relationships imply different expectations, and what is acceptable for a parent to do for a child – even an adult child – may not be so in reverse. Breaching these boundaries may cause embarrassment and require special techniques of social distancing. Parker found these structured inhibitions applied to spouse carers also, and no assumption should be made as to the easy extension of marital intimacy to other forms of physical intimacy (Parker 1993). The experience of providing personal care is also mediated by gender. Cross-gender tending of an intimate character threatens conventional expectations concerning what a man should see and touch in relation to a woman and vice versa. These cross-gender rules have an asymmetrical character to them. What men may do for women in relation to bodily contact is more highly constrained than women for men. This relates both to the ways in which men's and women's bodies are treated differently culturally, and the different roles of the sexes in the management of them. As a result, cross-gender tending appears to be more problematic when provided by males for females, and the intimate labour of personal care more associated with women than men.

Evidence from the study supported these broad conclusions concerning cultural assumptions. Men either found it more difficult to undertake cross-gender tending than women, or felt more justified in refusing to do it. Male carers were more likely to define specific boundaries around what they would or would not do. Several male carers, for example, said they would feel awkward and embarrassed if they had to bath their mother. Mr and Mrs Webb, who looked after their daughter, Dawn, who suffered from muscular atrophy, endorsed a clear division of labour, with the husband refusing to undertake personal care. As he explained:

> 'Not with a girl of thirty-odd years old, let's be honest . . . If it had been a lad it would have been the other way round, wouldn't it? . . . It would be embarrassing for Dawn and embarrassing for me.'

Mrs Otterburn, caring for her physically disabled daughter, similarly felt it would be impossible for her husband to undertake such tasks and was much concerned about who would deal with her daughter's incontinence if anything were to happen to her. The 'private' nature of these tasks meant the carer sometimes turned to the family for help rather than service practitioners. Mr Chappel, for example, arranged for his sister to bath his mother. Mrs Pearse felt she could not wash her husband's 'private parts' and therefore her son called once a week to give him a bath.

The second feature of personal care tasks is that they need to be performed on demand or at particular times. Tasks such as toileting and dressing, unlike housework or shopping, cannot be accumulated, but need to be undertaken immediately, as the need arises. Practitioners, however, find it difficult to provide a service on this basis. These are not problems that have a natural service shape.

Sometimes carers undertook personal care tasks where there was no obvious need for them to do so, mostly for their own convenience. Mr Chappel, for example, who cared for his disabled mother, commented: 'Well she can get there eventually, you know, if we've got time and leave her to it, but we mostly have to do it.' This could create a dilemma for the carer. Should they allow them to undertake these tasks to preserve their independence or should the carer take over because it was the easiest way of getting things done? For some carers, involvement with personal tending did not mean undertaking these tasks so much as supervising and directing the cared-for person. This was particularly so where there was some form of mental impairment. Mrs Chilton, for example, described how her husband, who had dementia, would sit in the bath for hours if she did not supervise him. In other cases the carer wanted to be on hand if anything went wrong. Mrs Leach looked after her chronically ill husband, and although he could bath himself she always kept an eye on him: 'Just to be on the safe side because with him having high blood pressure it's a bit dodgy.'

In these ways, carers could end up doing more than was immediately obvious from the disability of the cared-for person. How carers constructed their responsibilities was important in defining their experience of caring and with it their need for help. Service providers did not always define the situation in the same way.

The community nursing service was the main source of help cited by carers. The levels of assistance offered by the nursing service were, however, constrained and, as we shall see in Chapter 5, personal care was the classic 'grey area' of nursing practice. The home-help service, in both areas, although beginning to move towards offering personal care, did so only to a limited degree. Area I had a Crossroads Care Attendant scheme, but demand had been so great it was no longer accepting referrals, and none of the carers included in the study received this service. In Area II there was no comparable scheme. Bath aids and adaptations represented the most frequent, and often only, form of help.

Incontinence

Incontinence is one of the most stressful aspects of caring (Blannin 1987; Levin *et al.* 1989), and one that is stigmatizing for both carer and cared-for person (Mandelstrom 1981; Glew 1986; Norton 1986). Certainly, the experience of our sample suggested that carers found the condition embarrassing. Mr Richards, for example, felt that he could not invite friends back to the house because of his brother's incontinence. Incontinence is often hidden or underplayed because of embarrassment or a wish to protect the cared-for person, and carers did not always reveal the difficulties they faced. Sometimes the problem was only revealed when the cared-for person attended a day centre or some form of respite.

Incontinence also poses practical difficulties, creating extra laundry, ranging from soiled bed linen to the cared-for person's clothes. Mr Rose remarked that his line was always full of washing. Other difficulties included having to change the cared-for person, manage catheters or clear up after 'accidents'. Some carers found changing incontinence pads and managing colostomy bags particularly distasteful. Mrs Lloyds, for example, looked after her brain-damaged husband who had also had an ileostomy. He could not manage the bag himself, and she had to cope: 'It smells dreadful. It really is horrible, but I've got to get used to doing it, but sometimes it really knocks you sick.' Going on holiday posed problems since she had no means of disposing of the bags and they sometimes burst which was embarrassing and could, she feared, lead to their being asked to leave their accommodation. The first few days of the holiday would be spent searching for a disabled lavatory for their disposal; and no one had informed her that there were lists of these or that she could get a key to the ones that were locked.

Carers sometimes faced problems over attempts to restrict supplies. Mrs Lloyds had been told that she must reuse the bags and this intensified the unpleasant nature of the job:

> 'I'm supposed to reuse the bag. I'm supposed to squeeze it out of the bag and empty it in to a jug and pour it down the lavatory and then wipe the bag off at the bottom and seal it off and leave it on. They reckon you can use one bag for five days and it's absolutely impossible. You can't. He can't keep a bag on a full day. The longest he can keep a bag on is for four or five hours and then it's right brim full and it's coming unstuck.'

She had protested to her GP, who although sympathetic, explained that he was under pressure to keep down prescriptions. Mrs Lloyds, however, stood her ground:

> 'I look after him the best way I can . . . He's not going to be comfortable if he's in a mess. I'm not going to be happy. So I just insist on having the bags. I'm not extravagant with them.'

Knowledge of continence services were poor among carers. Few had received advice and many were unaware that pads could be supplied on the health service. Some carers only discovered this by accident, in Mrs Thomas's case when the nurse came to treat her son's injured eye, and in Mrs Whitcombe's when her daughter went on holiday with the Adult Training Centre. Some carers felt they were not given enough, and found the service inflexible in supplying more. Mrs Thomas and Mrs Otterburn both had to supplement their monthly allocation by buying pads privately. Mr Coney was particularly angry because he felt he had no control over his sister's incontinence. When the district nurse suggested he should cut down on the number of pads he was using he responded: 'But, I said: "Oh, she'll stop pooing once a day, she'll do it every other day now." Well what am I going to do in between?' The attendance of the cared-for person at a day or respite centre often made the situation worse since these institutions used pads without regard to the restrictions placed on the carer.

Both areas operated some form of continence service within community nursing, offering advice and support, as well as aids to assist in managing the condition. In practice, advice and support was variable. As we have seen, carers often remained unaware of the existence of help and sought their own solutions in the open market. The picture confirmed that of other work that suggests that the service is uncertain and often of poor quality (Briggs and Oliver 1985; Hunter *et al.* 1988).

Nursing tasks

The boundary between personal tending and nursing tasks is not a fixed one, and the ways in which it is constructed varies. From the community nursing perspective, the tension is between a definition in terms of the sorts of tasks that nurses undertake on the ward – the defining locus of nursing – which encompass forms of physical tending, and a rival definition that focuses on those tasks that require a trained nurse to perform them. Although both approaches are traditionally embodied in community nursing, pressure from acute hospital discharges have increasingly resulted in a definition of nursing tasks in terms of those requiring skilled input. These pressures have also resulted in attempts to co-opt carers into semi-medical areas through training them. From the carers' point of view, however, nursing tasks are constructed rather differently. Some carers regard personal care as itself a nursing activity. This was particularly so with men or where cross-gender tending produced embarrassment. Although some carers did undertake tasks like giving injections, changing dressings and supervising medication, many felt uneasy doing so and some refused, feeling it was beyond their competence and something that a nurse should do.

Household tasks

Some carers, particularly those who were themselves old, had difficulties with household tasks. In other cases the need for help with household chores arose less from physical incapacity than from the general stress of caring which meant that housework was just another source of stress. Mr Cooper, for example, cared for his wife who had dementia and was doubly incontinent. When asked about the worst aspect of caring, he replied:

> 'Well everything really, shopping, washing, ironing. You've got to do everything . . . I don't have a rest when she is away. I'm always doing something, doing jobs that I can't do.'

Other work has suggested that men and women ascribe different 'personal meanings' to housework, with women less likely to perceive help with these tasks as necessary or appropriate (Ramdas 1986; Levin *et al.* 1989). The experience of our sample bore this out. Ms Myers, for example, was insulted by the offer of a home help, interpreting it, despite the fact that she had influenza and was highly stressed, as a comment on the way she ran the house. Male carers, on the other hand, were less likely to interpret this form of help as a rebuke, and found it easier to accept. Some male carers did take on new activities, but others found this difficult, or at least expected help. Mr Marwood, for example, described housework as 'women's work' and, although capable of performing household tasks, felt entitled to help with them. For women, however, it was often the traditional male tasks that they found daunting. Mrs Lloyds, for example, described the struggles she had in trying to knock in a nail or drill a hole. The home-help service, modelled on the female domestic role, was of little use and there was no comparable service that could meet the need.

Behaviourial difficulties

Behaviour problems pose particular difficulties for carers, and have been associated with high levels of stress and with care collapse (Gilleard *et al.* 1984; Levin *et al.* 1989). The problems vary with different conditions and can, as we shall see in Chapters 7 and 8, be acute in relation to severe learning disabilities and certain forms of mental illness.

Here our concern is with the impact of dementia. The behaviourial difficulties faced by carers looking after an older person with confusion have been well described (Gilhooly 1982; Gilleard *et al.* 1984; Brook and Jestice 1986; Levin *et al.* 1989), and carers in the study faced a similar range of behaviourial and interpersonal problems. These included the inability of the cared-for person to converse normally, repetition, restlessness, unsafe acts such as forgetting to turn off the gas, wandering, not recognizing the carer, lack of purposeful activity, hitting out at the carer and disturbing their sleep. All were highly stressful for the carers. Mr Greig, looking after his mother who, as a result of dementia, suffered from 'extreme bouts of violence' and 'aggressive behaviour', explained: 'If the mood takes her she will just pick up a knife and go for me . . . She can be sitting quietly one minute and the next minute just go for me.' Mrs Chilton found her husband's night disturbance particularly difficult to cope with:

> 'Oh well he's up and down, up and down all night, and you're getting so bad tempered . . . I can't get any sleep. So I mean I've never yet, well, for the last three years had a sleep the night through.'

Changes in personality caused particular pain. Some carers described the acute sense of loss and bereavement this could produce. As Mrs Askew explained:

> 'It's like living with a stranger now . . . I just feel I'm living with somebody, it's not the man I married you see. It's not Tom, it's not me, we're just two different people.'

Often the cared-for person could not co-operate in their care, and their inability to respond in a meaningful way depressed carers. Not being recognized or thanked was especially painful.

The behaviourial difficulties associated with dementia are among the hardest for services to address directly. Service provision cannot reverse the dementing process or recover the relationship that has been destroyed. Medication, information and respite were the main sources of help. Medication was provided by psychogeriatricians or, occasionally, general practitioners. Day-hospital staff and community nurses were often important in bringing these needs to the attention of a doctor. Mr Dilley, for example, described how the insistent talking of his wife, who suffered from dementia, gave him 'tremendous headaches' and often prevented him from getting a night's sleep. The carer mentioned this to the district nurse, who brought it to the attention of the consultant, who prescribed 'liquid medicine' which 'calmed' her down.

Information and advice were potentially available from all the service providers with whom the carer was in contact, although it was rare for them to receive systematic advice or counselling on how to handle behaviourial problems. Carer support groups were a useful source of information and advice. Support groups also offered the opportunity to talk to others and exchange advice. Day centres and hospitals provided a welcome break, but appeared to play only a minor part in trying to modify the person's behaviour. Few carers saw the centres in these terms, though Mrs Gilling whose husband had post-stroke dementia felt that his behavioural problems, which arose in part in her view from his frustration and boredom, were alleviated by the stimulation that he got at the day hospital.

Restrictedness

Restrictedness is the term we employ for an experience that is central to the lives of most carers. At its simplest it represents the degree to which the carer is unable to leave the cared-for person, but it also encapsulates the wider ways in which care-giving limits and constrains the carer's life. The carer literature has described at length the feelings of frustration, boredom and claustrophobia that often accompany caring (Robinson and Thurner 1979; Lovelock 1985; Stephens and Christiansen 1986; Bebbington *et al.* 1986). Restrictedness can be constructed in three ways. In its simplest, concrete, form it arises from the limitations imposed by the need to do things for the cared-for person, such as toileting, or to be with them to ensure their physical safety. The time the person could be left alone varied, and for some carers, particularly those looking after someone with dementia, the restrictedness was total.

For many carers, however, it was not so much concrete tasks of caring that restricted them, as a general anxiety about what might happen in their absence. This second form of restrictedness was more open to interpretation and although there seemed no 'objective reason' why the cared-for person could not be left, the carer was ill at ease when away and tried to limit such occasions as much as possible. The experience of Mrs Quigley illustrates this point in its most extreme form. Her son, Mark, had suffered from Crohn's disease for 15 years. His severe bowel problems meant that he was afraid to move far from the lavatory, and spent long hours there. The illness preyed on his mind to the extent he became a recluse, never leaving the house. He became depressed and made a suicide attempt. Mrs Quigley became fearful of leaving him on his own:

> 'I used to dread going back home . . . in case I found something. You know I just did not know what I was going to walk into. I thought, "Oh he's all right". You know my stomach would be churning.'

As a result she stopped going out in the evening, and tried to ensure he was alone as little as possible during the day. The case illustrates three important features. First, certain situations are potentially so rebuking to the carers that they affect decisions out of proportion to the likelihood of their happening. Second, this form of restrictedness, resulting from fears that are private and scarcely ever articulated, is particularly easy for service providers to miss. Third, the problems of restrictedness may not always appropriately be met by respite. Sometimes what is needed is a new perspective on the situation, and sensitive intervention from practitioners can help provide this.

Finally, some carers suffer from shared or secondary restrictedness when the limits placed on the person they looked after also affect their lives. This was particularly evident among spouse carers who did not want to pursue an independent social life. Mrs Stenton whose husband had muscular sclerosis remarked that caring had not so much affected *her* social life as *their* social life. Mrs Gorst, whose husband had a severe lung disease, could no longer cope with smoky or confined spaces, and although he encouraged her to go out on her own, she felt awkward about leaving him: 'Well actually I have gone out and I have been so ill while I've been out, thinking where I am. I feel guilty.'

In the construction of restrictedness the legitimacy of the rival activity is of central importance. Thus it was clear that even carers who look after someone who 'could not be left' did on occasion risk a brief absence, but only where the need was unquestioned. Vital food shopping fell into this category. Thus Mr Chilton, caring for a wife with dementia said:

> 'I've never left her on her own. Only for five minutes when I've been going down the shop on the corner for a couple of pies, she's been sat down there and gone to sleep you see. I never leave her at all. I'm frightened of leaving her.'

Such snatched outings are often accompanied by considerable stress, and can go badly wrong, as Ms McAllen recounted when she fell on the pavement outside the shop injuring her leg badly. As she was lying in pain in the hospital, all she could think about was what was happening to her mother with dementia left locked in the house.

Certain social activities carry some legitimacy. Thus one carer accepted overnight respite but only in order to attend regular MENCAP meetings. Attending church was another form of legitimate personal activity, as was paid employment, at least for some. What clearly had a low level of legitimacy for carers was enjoying themselves. This was not something that carers seemed to be able to make the psychic space to do. A number of carers described how they were on edge all the time that they were out. While this was tolerable for shopping, it clearly made impossible any sense of relaxation or enjoyment. Time away from the cared-for person was never fully their time, but compromised by the presence of the cared-for person at home.

Carers used the time away from the person they looked after for practical tasks, such as shopping, or for some modest form of relaxation and social recreation. Mrs Reeves, who looked after her disabled husband, for example, could contrast the situation before her husband attended a day centre and after:

> 'I was running round the shops . . . and I was back as soon as I could, because I was afraid of something happening while I was out. Now when he

is at [name of day centre] as soon as I wave cheerio at the van, I don't worry about him, because I know he is in good hands . . . I can get into [name of town] and wander round, relax a bit.'

The ways in which restrictedness is constructed has consequences for service support. Visibility can be a problem. In general service providers are best at recognizing the first, concrete, form of restrictedness, imposed by the need to do things for the cared-for person. Where it arises from general anxieties or shared restrictedness the problem is less visible and the service provider can remain unaware of its consequences for the carer. Second, the restrictions imposed by caring can destroy the carer's social life to the extent that the offer of respite has limited appeal. If you no longer have friends, outings can be lonely and dispiriting on your own. Mrs Chivers, caring for her disabled husband said:

'I want company. You can do lots of things on your own, but it gets to the point where you are lonely . . . I think that is the worst part of it – caring for people – the loneliness.'

Spouse carers faced a particular dilemma. They often expressed a need to get away from the claustrophobia of the other person's constant company, and yet the person they most wanted to go out with was their spouse. Mrs Chivers who had been offered respite for her husband to allow her to go on a holiday, remarked: 'But I'd like to go with him. That's the point. You see, he goes somewhere, when I go somewhere, we are not together.' Untying these links can be disturbing. Wanting relief can seem disloyal to your partner. As Parker (1993) notes, relief from caring actually threatens the basis of why you are together and married. Building up a separate life can threaten the relationship. And yet without such elements of independence and autonomy, effective relief is impossible.

Last, the restrictedness imposed by caring can itself erode self-confidence in ways that undermine the carer's capacity to accept relief. Both Mrs Gorst and Mrs Harrison had on occasion become fearful of going out, and avoided meeting people. Carers sometimes so make their lives around caring that any attempt to offer relief itself becomes disturbing. We shall explore this further in Chapter 8 when we discuss carers who have become engulfed by their role.

Carers sometimes called on the support of their families to give them a break. Not all, however, had such support and many carers found that caring eroded their social networks in ways that made it hard to call on such support. Where the cared-for person was young, as we shall see in relation to learning disabilities and mental health problems, carers were sometimes able to pursue educational and work training opportunities for them, partly in order to get a break for themselves. For the other client groups the sources of relief were more limited, centring on day care and respite. We shall discuss their impact in Chapter 6.

The need to talk

Caring can be a lonely and isolating experience. It disrupts social networks and cuts people off from human contact (Ungerson 1987; Parker 1990a). Many carers need a chance to talk, and this is particularly so where the cared-for person can no longer sustain a conversation (Levin *et al.* 1989). Mrs Gilling felt that the most difficult aspect of caring for her mother with dementia was the loneliness. Mrs Chivers, who looked after her physically disabled husband, agreed:

> 'It does everybody good to have a good chat . . . Sometimes I sit here and think I'm going mad. I must be going mad . . . I felt as though I was cut off from everything.'

Some carers needed to 'let off steam', usually during a crisis. Ms Myers, for example, telephoned her sister-in-law when the situation got too much: 'I scream down the phone at Jackie when it gets too much, poor Jackie.'

Many carers simply wanted someone to acknowledge and value what they did. Mrs Leach, who looked after her chronically ill husband, remarked:

> 'If someone just came, now and again, to talk to you, you know, to let you know there was someone out there even if it was only once every couple of months, just to let you know there was someone there, knowing your position and thinking about you.'

Talking about the situation could also reinforce the carers' perceptions of themselves as such, helping to establish their right to think of themselves and their needs. Some carers used talking to others as a means of coming to terms with the cared-for person's disability and with it their own situation. Not all carers wanted to dwell on this. Mr Cooper, for example, saw no point in talking; it solved nothing and was a waste of time. Some carers wanted to talk about something different from caring for once, and to have an opportunity to be recognized as something other than a carer.

Carers looked for support from a number of sources. In the absence of mental impairment, carers could usually talk to the person they looked after. Many did so, although several felt inhibited because they did not want to upset the cared-for person or make them feel guilty. Mrs Leach, for example, found it difficult to talk to her disabled husband. She often had 'a little cry', but never in front of him: 'Well he would just think it was him.'

The people that carers most commonly talked to were other family members. Families – particularly grandchildren – could also provide an alternative home-based interest for the carer besides caring. Several carers, however, could not talk to other family members. Mrs Ashworth, for example, could not discuss her worries about their son with her husband because he hated to see her upset. Several carers felt they could not talk to sons and daughters because they did not wish to burden them. Mrs Leach, whose children visited regularly, did not discuss the situation with them because she wanted to hide the full extent of her husband's disability. The carer could also be inhibited by tensions within the family concerning the cared-for person. In some cases this was made worse by the carer's unexpressed resentment over the lack of support offered by other family members. Ms McAllen knew that her sister and niece thought that her mother should go into a home, and this limited how much she felt she could say to them.

Besides family, the opportunity for contact outside the home was limited, and many carers experienced difficulty in maintaining close relationships. Mrs Reeves was conscious how her husband's disability had lost them friends:

> 'Well, it's strange. We thought we had lots of friends. But when this happened it was just as though there was a plague on the house . . . Do they think we are going to ask them to do things for us? . . . Or are they embarrassed, you know, because they can do things we can't?'

Several carers expressed a reluctance to talk to friends even when they had an opportunity to do so. Mr Dilley did not want to be seen as a 'moaner'. Experience made Mrs Reeves aware of the dangers of confiding in someone else:

> 'And I was telling my friend, and I said, "Do you know, I don't want to go home tonight" . . . And she just looked at me and said: "Well, we've all got our troubles, Ethel." And if she had gone wham and smacked me across the face, she couldn't have hurt me more. And after that, I thought never again will I tell anybody. And if I meet anybody when I'm out and they say, "How's Peter?," "Oh he's just the same," "And how are you,?" "Oh bearing up, you know." And I thought never ever, 'cos it was such a shock.'

Most carers preferred to talk to family members and friends rather than service practitioners. This does not mean, however, that service providers were not relevant in this area. Some carers had no one else to talk to, and home helps were particularly valued as a source of company and conversation. Carer support groups offered a chance to share experiences, let off steam and find companionship. Any service contact potentially offers the carer a chance to unburden and talk about the situation. Several carers found service providers supportive in letting them talk and express their feelings, but there was no systematic structure that allowed for such contacts, and they depended on individual practice. Some carers recognized the *ad hoc* nature of these contacts and would have perferred something more structured, particularly something that did not require them to put themselves forward. Carers were diffident in their dealings with service providers, and needed encouragement and active permission to talk. They were reluctant to take the initiative themselves. An important part of the need to talk concerns negotiating what has happened in your life. Information about the cared-for person's condition and its likely course can be vital, and can, for example, allow the carer to perceive the distressing behaviour in terms of a medical condition rather than the person themselves. As we shall see, however, such information was not always easy to come by.

The financial consequences of caring

The financial costs of caring can be considerable, and have been documented by Glendinning and others (Baldwin 1985; McLaughlin 1991; Glendinning 1992). Caring affects people's ability to participate fully in the labour market, and can isiderable impact on family's earnings; the average gross earnings for all .vith children are 9 per cent higher for men and 7 per cent higher for women than those found among parents with disabled children (Smyth and Robus 1989). Loss of earnings, however, is only one facet of the financial aspects of caring, and is compounded by higher day-to-day living expenses (Baldwin 1985; Glendinning 1992). Among the causes of extra expenditure mentioned in the study were clothing, bedding, laundry, heating, transport, special food and diets, housing and housing adaptations, repairs to the house and furniture, and aids to mobility and daily living.

Carers tend to have low incomes, and many rely on the benefit system for support. There is only one state benefit explicitly designed for carers: Invalid Care Allowance (ICA). Its purpose is to compensate for loss of employment, but its impact is complicated by interactions with other forms of income support, and few carers claim it. In 1989, for example, of those providing 20 hours or more of care a week, 10 per cent received the benefit (McLaughlin 1991). In addition to ICA there is a range of benefits paid to the cared-for person which were drawn upon by the carer. Sometimes this resulted in a situation where the carer was financially dependent on the cared-for person, and the interrelationship of the carer's and the cared-for person's incomes could cause disagreement over who controlled the money (Hirst 1984, 1990; McLaughlin 1991; Glendinning 1992).

At the time of the fieldwork other benefits included attendance allowance, mobility allowance, invalidity benefit and severe disablement allowance, as well as general benefits such as income support. Since then there have been a number of changes. These do not, however, affect the general issues discussed here, for our focus is not on the adequacy of the benefit system as such, so much as on the problems carers faced in accessing it and the sources of help they found in doing so. Carers identified various factors that inhibited them from claiming benefits. First was lack of information. This is confirmed by other work. Amongst the carers interviewed, as in other work (Kerr 1982; Ritchie and Mathews 1982; Graham 1984), knowledge of the benefit system was poor and many had little idea about whether they were eligible. They often found out about benefits in an *ad hoc* way, through a leaflet in the post office or a chance conversation. These informal sources meant that knowledge was acquired in a hit-and-miss fashion, and carers often did not discover the full range of their entitlement. Sometimes they were held back from applying by mistaken ideas about benefits. One carer believed that attendance allowance was available only if the cared-for person was incontinent, while another thought the cared-for person would need to be bedridden. Sometimes service providers added to the confusion by giving wrong advice. This is perhaps understandable given the complexities of the benefit system, but it created difficulties for carers. Mr Howland, for example, was told by his GP that he could not claim mobility allowance because he did not have a car. Carers also assumed that previous contact with a service provider meant they would have been informed of their full entitlement. Mrs Thomas, whose son had a learning disability, had previously contacted a social worker for help in claiming attendance allowance. She presumed that the social worker would have told her if she was entitled to further benefits, and it came as a surprise, therefore, to discover she could claim mobility allowance.

Carers found the benefit system confusing and complex. They were rarely aware of the detailed rules that applied to the receipt of benefits. Few had any idea which benefits were means tested, or would credit them with National Insurance contributions. Dealing with the social security system was just an additional complication in their already demanding role as a carer. As Mrs Stenton explained: 'You can do without the aggravation. When you've got enough problems as it is you can do without it.'

Appealing was an added source of anxiety – one that could be humiliating. Mrs Reeves, who looked after her physically disabled husband, described her feelings after their appeal for attendance allowance was refused:

> 'We've never been so shattered. We came home and we both felt like putting . . . well we have not got a gas oven, otherwise we might have done. And he [the doctor] as good as said it was all in his mind.'

Some did appeal successfully, and found service providers who would support them in the sometimes rather tortuous process of doing so.

Employment

Caring affects the ability of carers to take paid employment (Baldwin 1985; Joshi 1987; McLaughlin 1991; Glendinning 1992). They are less likely to be in employment than comparable non-carers (Green 1988; Martin and Wright 1988; Parker and Lawton 1990b), and those who attempt to combine caring with work face reduction of hours, fewer opportunities for overtime, restricted career development and loss of pension rights (Hyman 1977; EOC 1980; Nissel and Bonnerjea 1982; Lewis and Meredith 1988). Beyond this, the impact of caring on paid employment varies between different disability groups, mainly because of differences in the carers' ages and household circumstances (Parker 1990a). The carer's gender and marital status also mediate the impact. Lewis and Meredith (1988) found that single daughters were particularly reluctant to give up paid work; some women are able to become 'career carers' because their husbands maintain them financially (Glendinning 1992).

The importance of work for carers is not simply financial: it also offers a break from caring and a source of company (Gilhooly 1982; Glendinning 1983; Parker 1993). Employment has a legitimacy that is not accorded to other activities outside the home. Mrs Leach, for example, who was otherwise closely confined by her husband's demands and her own distress, did manage to escape for a few hours a day to go to work. The complex way in which employment could sustain caring was illustrated in the case of Mr Ensbury, a single man in his late sixties, who was caring for a mother with severe dementia. He used his income from his pharmacy to pay for private nurses to cover for him during the day. He would have liked to retire and sell the business, but this would have meant that he no longer had the income, nor the reason to pay for substitute care, and would be forced to stay at home twenty-four hours a day. He needed to work to generate the income to allow him to work and thus escape from the situation.

A number of carers in the study, particularly spouse carers, had given up work to care. Often this happened suddenly as an immediate reaction to the onset of disability. At this point they were rarely in contact with service providers who might allow them to reflect on the decision or discuss available options. The effects of caring were not confined to giving up or losing a job. Some carers had had to turn down opportunities of promotion because they could not go away on training courses or because they would involve working full time. As Mrs Hobson commented:

> 'The strain would have been too much. So there's no way you could hold down a full-time job . . . I was upset because it was the job I always wanted.'

Caring can also restrict long-term opportunities for re-entering the labour market. Several carers would have liked to get back into the labour market but felt that their lack of recent work experience excluded them.

About a third of the carers interviewed were in some form of employment. Few, however, sustained conventional jobs; the majority were either in part-time work or some form of employment which allowed them to control their work environments, such as running a market stall or working as a bookkeeper from home. Those carers who worked in more conventional settings had to rely on the goodwill of their employers, or help from other kin. Mrs Addy praised her employer:

> 'She knows I've got me dad living with me and she's quite good . . . We've discussed me dad, that sometimes I might have to come to work late, things like that, and she, you know, she just accepts this.'

In general, those carers who worked did so by virtue of their own initiative rather than through the support of services. Some carers drew on the help of family and neighbours. Those who did use services like day care had to fit their employment around provision rather than the other way round. Day care is not designed to allow carers to engage in paid work, and the number of days available, the short hours, and the uncertain transport limit its relevance.

Housing

Although housing forms part of the environment of caring, it has received little attention as such. The role of housing in community care is itself a neglected topic, although one that has begun to be addressed more recently (Wertheimer 1989; Mackintosh *et al.* 1990; Oldman 1990, 1991), and there is as yet no systematic exploration of housing issues in relation to informal care. Housing did however feature as an issue in the carer interviews.

In general, the carers in the study were well housed. Area I in particular had had a long and creditable tradition of public housing, and this was reflected in the situation of carers. It was only in a minority of cases that problems arose, and they tended to occur among carers of people with physical disabilities or where the carer or cared-for person was elderly, reflecting housing problems general to these groups. The main difficulties that had a carer dimension related to poor-quality housing, inappropriate accommodation, the need for space, or issues arising from tenure and inheritance.

Poor-quality housing can make the tasks of caring more burdensome. Mr Cooper, for example, looked after his wife who was doubly incontinent. Their house had no downstairs toilet, and because his wife had mobility difficulties, she found it difficult to get upstairs. He had had a sani-loo fitted in a cupboard but it was awkward to manoeuvre her into it, it needed to be emptied, and his health was also poor. Inappropriate housing can also increase the tasks of caring by impeding the independence of the cared-for person. Mrs Arne and her daughter had been re-housed at the top of a steep slope, and this meant she could no longer get out to shop and meet people. Many carers were themselves elderly or in poor health and found their accommodation inappropriate to their needs. Mrs Hobson, who had a bad heart and was almost blind, cared for her son, who was diagnosed as schizophrenic. The flat they shared was small and up a flight of stairs that she found difficult to manage. She asked if it would be possible for her to move with her son into the housing association accommodation that was being planned to provide community support for people with mental health problems. She was told that if a double flat came up she would be considered. This for her would be the ideal. It was unlikely, however, that this would be actively supported by psychiatric staff, since their aim was to increase her son's independence and not underwrite what they saw as her over-involvement and reliance on him. Here issues of caring, housing and the transfer to independence became interlinked.

Issues of housing touch on the ways in which carers organize their lives spatially. Carers use space as a part of their coping strategies, and it can have symbolic as well as material significance relating to the frustration and claustrophobia that some carers experience in sharing limited accommodation, particularly with someone who is mentally disturbed and with whom they can no longer have a normal conversation. It is difficult to distance yourself psychically when you cannot get away physically. Mrs Todd's husband could no longer go upstairs and when she was angry with him she went there to get away. She said she would never move to a bungalow because of this. As we shall see in Chapter 9, such use of space can be important in underwriting a more boundary-setting approach to caring.

Finally, housing plays a major role in capital accumulation. Many carers, however, felt angry at what they perceived as their exclusion from these benefits. Mrs Hewson believed that had it not been for caring for their disabled daughter they would have been owner-occupiers with all the freedom and financial advantage that implied. Mr Coney believed that the extension they had had built to their council house meant that they were no longer eligible under the right to buy legislation. The carer who had the most to lose in terms of housing capital was Ms Myers, a single women in her thirties caring for a mother with dementia. The house was owned by her mother, and Ms Myers was anxious that she might become homeless if her mother were to go into residential care. Her social worker had assured her that she would be re-housed, but this did not meet her anxieties about losing both the capital value of the house and, as she saw it, her only chance, as a single women without good employment prospects, of owning her own house. When asked if the issue of the house had made any difference to her decision to keep her mother living with her she said: 'Yes it does. In a way, I mean, they adopted me to give me a better life and all that, she's saved up, and all that she's got she wants to be mine. I can't make her see it might not be.'

In seeking remedies to housing difficulties, carers had access to the same sources as the rest of the population. Prior patterns of tenure largely determined their options: owner-occupiers looking to the market, and local authority tenants to the housing department or housing associations. Both sought help from local authorities with adaptations to their houses.

Among those looking for more suitable accommodation, the main problem was one of availability. Mrs Askew, for example, had put her name down to move into sheltered housing three years ago but had been told it was a question of waiting for someone to die. Even when a carer had moved to specialist or sheltered housing they could still experience problems. Sheltered accommodation, in particular, often provided limited space. Mrs Chilton had recently moved to a one-bedroom purpose-built bungalow as a solution to her previous housing problems. She, however, found her new accommodation small, and sharing the bedroom with her husband, who had dementia, was a strain:

> 'It is terrible in bed. I never get a night's sleep . . . I should have stuck out for a two-bedroomed one really, because I could do with a bedroom in my own right now really.'

Not all carers sought a solution to their accommodation problems through specialist housing. Some preferred to adapt or extend their homes. When carers pursued this option, the main impression was one of frustration, delay and poor-quality work, though alleviated on occasion by good professional support. The case of Mr Bowd illustrates some of the difficulties carers encountered. A man of fifty caring for his wife who had muscular sclerosis, he approached social services to ask to have handrails and a stair lift installed:

> 'The women there started laughing and said: "Oh no, things don't happen like that, it's got to go through. And it will be two years before you get it." I said, "Forget it love."'

He decided to buy his own lift. It cost £300 second-hand, and he paid for its installation by doing odd jobs for the electrician and joiner. Twelve months later, social services got back in touch. They did an assessment but would not refund him the cost of the lift. He retorted that they would have had to come and assess him for a new back if he had not acted 'because my back would have gone lifting and carrying her up and down stairs'.

He had seen the name of the disabled living centre in the paper where it was asking for donations, and he and his wife went down there. At first they were told that they needed to be referred but he persuaded them to let them in. They selected a number of items. He chose this route partly because he wanted to shortcut the endless bureaucracy and delay that seemed to be involved with

social services; but he also felt that he could get hold of bette
attractive items.

Relations with social services eventually took a turn for occupational therapist got in touch with him. He had eff social services:

> 'We was happily buying our own and doing our own thing, and th two and a half years of having a disabled sticker, I got a visit from [name]. She said, "You have got a disabled sticker and you know that is all you've got, we don't know anything about you."'

He was delighted with her help. She arranged for social services to take over the maintenance of the lift, and brought a number of useful aids and adaptations. He said she was very knowledgable and generally 'smashing'. He would call on her as his first point of contact.

Mr Bowd felt he had learned a lot as a result of his experiences. He would not now buy his stair lift. He would wait for the assessment and

> '... then shout like hell ... We have learnt in a way that if you start shouting and you create, the more you create the more you get. If you just get on with it then nobody bothers ... I am now wiser ... I am learning the game, which in a lot of instances I think it is.'

His account was not an isolated one, and its main themes recur in other interviews: the delays, the incomprehensibility of bureaucracy, the poor quality of the equipment, and above all the need to shout.

Information

Lack of information was repeatedly emphasized as a problem by carers. They faced the classically circular difficulty of not knowing what it was that they did not know until they had found it out. Mrs Radband commented that it was difficult to think about what she needed because she did not know what was available. Several carers recounted how it was only after many years of service contact that they discovered, by chance, some useful piece of information. Many carers felt it was up to them to find out what was available. Mrs Webb commented:

> 'You don't know what you can get and no one comes to you. They don't really come to you and say look I can do this or you can have that ... If you don't scream for anything they'll leave you alone and that's it you know.'

Some carers took a more cynical view about the lack of information from service providers. As Mr Coney commented: 'They're there to save money, not to give it out.'

The fragmented nature of support received by carers meant there was no single focus from which they could obtain systematic information. The service system is not a system at all, but a series of discrete services or even of discrete service encounters. No single service provider had a comprehensive view. Carers ght information from the most accessible service providers, but these were ɔt always the most appropriate. General practitioners, for example, were often the carer's only contact, and were asked about a wide range of subjects from benefits to help with aids and adaptations. Understandably, they rarely had this depth of knowledge, and were not always active in referring on to other sources.

Not surprisingly, what carers repeatedly said they wanted was a single accessible source of comprehensive advice – someone who would tell them about their full entitlement and not wait for them to ask. As Mrs Reeves said, 'I think there should be someone that will call, if it is only once a month . . . Someone who would advise you on practically anything.' Some carers recognized, however, that there was a gap between acquiring information and obtaining help. Mrs Trolle commented: 'Like I say, you can get books that say you can apply for this and you can get that, but when you come to try, it's a different thing, isn't it?' As we saw in Chapter 2, the services to which carers relate tend to be discretionary in character and this factor is reinforced by the ambiguous position of carers within the service system. As a result, it is difficult for carers to obtain clear information about eligibility and availability. We shall return to this problem in Chapter 11.

Chapter 4 *SOCIAL SERVICES*

In Chapters 4 to 6, we explore the responses of service providers to carers starting with those located in social service departments, moving on to those in the health sector and concluding with services in mixed settings. The pattern of service response is largely determined by the client-group status of the cared-for person and we concentrate here on the carers of younger people with physical disabilities and of older people with physical and mental disabilities. Service responses to people caring for someone with learning disabilities or mental health problems are discussed in Chapters 7 and 8.

Social workers

Social workers are the dominant and senior profession in the social services department, although not all clients will see one and many will be assisted by other staff. As key figures in the mobilization of support within the social services department, they occupy a parallel position to that of GPs in the health sector, albeit with important differences, particularly in regard to their location within a line management structure, their status and their lesser degree of professionalization (Huntingdon 1981). In the past their role has often been presented in terms of the case work activities that carry the greatest prestige within the profession. Increasingly, however, they are seen as the creators and managers of packages of care. It is in relation to both these roles that they are significant for carers.

During the 1980s there was a move within the organization of social services departments away from generic or intake/long-term models towards client-group specialism (Challis and Ferlie 1986, 1987, 1988) and both the areas in the study had been reorganized on this basis. Even where social work has been generic, there has been a long-established informal specialism whereby trained social workers predominantly deal with child-care cases, and work with older and physically disabled people has been left to untrained social workers. As a result, carers are largely in contact with untrained social workers (distinguished here as assistant social workers), and it was only in the more complex cases, usually involving interpersonal conflict or the transition into residential care, that carers came in contact with a trained social worker.

Social workers do similar things for carers as they do for elderly and disabled people (Rowlings 1981; Barclay 1982), and most of their work is concerned with marshalling practical help. However, they also have a potentially important role to play in talking to carers, allowing them to ventilate their feelings and share their experiences. Of all the practitioners involved with carers, social workers had the strongest tradition of counselling; social workers did provide carers with support of this kind, though contacts were in general short term, and it was rare for carers to be able to express their feelings over time. Social workers also have an important role to play in the process of negotiation. As we shall see, social workers were more aware of potential conflicts of interest between the carer and the cared-for person than other practitioners, and in certain cases were actively involved in negotiating these. Social workers were also aware of the barriers that might prevent carers from accepting help, and were sometimes involved in persuading them to overcome these. The predominantly short-term nature of their contact, however, meant that they were not in the same position to pursue this over time as were some other practitioners like district nurses or day-care managers. Occasionally, social workers, usually assistant social workers, did things of a practical nature for carers such as driving them down to the chemist, or making snacks when they were ill. These activities were undertaken unofficially, and were not endorsed by social work managers.

Most carers come into the orbit of a social worker as a result of the referral of the person they look after. Hospital discharge was one of the commonest routes into contact, particularly for carers of older people. Not all wards had a social work input, however, and carers of people with medical or surgical conditions sometimes lost out at this point. Where carers self-referred, it was usually for a defined form of help such as aids. A small number of carers came into contact with a social worker as a result of being referred back from services such as home care, day care and respite, all of which had a clear sense of a boundary beyond which their expertise and practice did not go; if a situation became very fraught, the case would be handed to a social worker. Typically in relation to carers, these were cases where the situation appeared to be near collapse or where the carer was voicing an intention to give up.

The issues raised by caring are at the heart of social work, relating as they do to the social environment of the client, to interpersonal difficulties and to the functioning of families. Not surprisingly, therefore, social workers appeared to incorporate carers to a greater degree in their practice than did other service providers, though the differences should not be exaggerated. Most social workers were familiar with the term 'carer', and applied it to the majority of cases in the study. Despite this greater awareness of the issue, the predominant response remained that of regarding carers as a form of *resource.* They were recognized as an important part of the support system of clients. To this degree they were more visible than was the case with, for example, hospital consultants for whom carers scarcely existed in professional terms, but it was a form of visibility that still made them ancillary to the needs of the person for whom they cared.

The more straightforward the case and the less trained the social worker, the greater the inclination to regard the carer in these limited terms. The organizational focus of the social worker's job could also encourage a particularly narrow remit, as for example with the social worker who worked for a housing charity and had been involved with Mr Plumb, an elderly man caring for his wife who had severe mental health problems. At his request, she had arranged for both of them to enter residential care in order to secure Mrs Plumb's support after his possible death (he had a heart problem). The social worker regarded the decision as relatively straightforward, and was much less concerned than was the community psychiatric nurse with its implications for him. The focus of her work, being on those housed by the charity and thus only on single elderly people or couples, meant that she was less attuned to carer issues than might have been the case had she worked in a wider context with a greater range of caring relationships, and she did not, in common with some other practitioners, associate caring with the situation of spouses.

Despite their primary focus on carers as resources, social workers were able to shift relatively easily in the more acute cases into regarding carers as *co-clients* who had needs themselves that the social worker should recognize and try to address. By contrast, the *co-worker* model was rarely employed, despite its superficial appeal to social work values. This endorses other work that has suggested that interweaving between formal and informal sources of help is difficult to achieve and contains inherent instabilities that arise from the different bases of the two forms of help (Froland 1981; Bayley 1982; Bulmer 1986; Twigg 1990a). Where the co-worker model did form the basis of practice, it was associated with certain relationships or client groups – with siblings or with those suffering from a congenital disability. (We will explore these patterns further in Chapter 9.) In these cases, social workers did attempt to work alongside, and with, the carer.

Most social work contact with carers focused around the assessment and allocation of a limited package of services; the majority of carers were only in contact with a social worker as part of their route to respite, day care or other practical help. Contact of this nature produced many plaudits; carers were full of praise for the help that social workers had given them. Thus Mrs Askew, who was caring for her husband with dementia remarked: 'I couldn't be more grateful.' Mr Rose commented that the social worker 'got things moving . . . he always found places for getting Dad away'. Ms Arne was similarly impressed: 'the social worker really kicked himself into gear'. These comments parallel the conclusions of other work that suggests that social workers are valued by their clients and are effective when they aim at modest and realistic goals (Sinclair *et al.* 1990).

As with other professional workers, the most significant source of implicit policy for social workers was professional training. The issues raised by carers were seen as the meat and drink of social work, so that although they recognized that carers as a group had risen to greater policy prominence in recent years, the questions they raised were regarded as sufficiently fundamental as always to have been an integral element in their professional training. As we have noted, however, the majority of social workers in contact with carers were untrained, and for this group the culture of the office and the shared assumptions of the team were a particularly important source of implicit policy. One assistant social worker explained how she had received no training in regard to carers as such: 'If you've got any problems, you ask round among your colleagues.' Another, commenting on the role of gender in allocation for carers described how her views had developed through such daily interchanges:

> 'I think unless you've been to college . . . I don't know, but I used to think that the woman was the one to do the caring, and if the man has to do it, you think, what a shame, he shouldn't have to do it. I am changing a little bit because I work with a team that is very much that way [i.e. in favour of equality].'

Social workers also drew on their own assumptive worlds when talking about their response to carers. The less-formally trained they were, the more they did so. In general, however, they made fewer direct appeals to 'common sense' or other shared understandings than did home help organizers or community nurses.

In regard to official policy, the majority of formal policy statements, both in the authorities studied and nationally, relate to child care; social work with elderly and disabled people largely takes place within the traditions of the activity rather than an explicit policy framework. Though there had been moves in both areas (particularly Area II) towards greater definition, the results of this at the time of the fieldwork had not reached the front line; in neither area was there a developed formal policy in relation to social work with carers.

It was not clear that social workers were operating any implicit priority system in allocating help to carers, beyond the general one of responding to those who put themselves forward. A small number of carers voiced the view that social workers only really responded if the carer was 'on the brink', and about to collapse. Mrs Webb, caring for a disabled daughter, commented: 'If you don't scream for anything, they'll leave you alone and that's it.' It was a view shared by Mr Coney caring for his multiply disabled sister:

> 'See, they have a system here, whereas if they think you're coping, or know you're coping I should say, they don't come and see you. They wait for you to go and see them.'

Certainly we had cases where social work intervention had only been mobilized as a result of a crisis. Thus Ms Myers, in the wake of influenza and depression, had hit her mother and the disclosure of this had resulted in the social worker organizing help and offering her quite considerable personal support. In the case of Ms Arne, caring for her very elderly adoptive mother, relations had deteriorated to the point where her mother had thrown her out. She rang social services. The duty social worker spent some time talking to her and a second social worker arranged various forms of help for her mother. Though she was impressed, she was critical of the fact that no help had been offered before the crisis:

> 'Nothing was ever done to help her at all, or ease any pressure on her, and then when I left, things seemed like . . . I don't know, I was quite stunned

actually . . . like maybe the fact that they had to get their finger out, now that she's actually on her own . . . Why were they waiting for me to leave before they did it. They say budgets are tight . . . all of a sudden within a few weeks the earth will move and things will get going. That's quite hypocritical, because I think obviously, certainly the services were there and it's only really that I wasn't that changed it.'

It was certainly the case that her leaving, like Ms Myers hitting her mother, had precipitated social work support, though it was not clear in either case that support had *only* resulted from the crisis. In large measure social workers responded to those cases that reached them, and did not operate a system that demanded crisis to justify support.

What was perhaps more significant in these two cases was the role of cultural expectations on behalf of the social workers concerning age, independence and a 'normal life'. Ms Arne was in her mid-twenties, caring for an adoptive mother in her eighties, and it was clear that both the social workers involved saw the case as much in terms of intergenerational conflict and the transition to adulthood as they did of caring. In Ms Myers' case, the extended social work involvement had resulted from a wish to increase her independence from her mother and from the engulfing caring situation. The social worker tried to enable her to have what she thought a single woman 34-year-old would want; and to this end, she tried to encourage her social contacts, improve her appearance, and raise her self-esteem. She arranged five-day-a-week day care so Ms Myers could go on courses that might lead her back into employment. But after a period of some months, she came to see that she was working towards goals that Ms Myers did not want: 'She used to block every effort that I made.' She withdrew regular contact, leaving it up to her to call when she needed her. It was clear however that the factor that had mediated the initial response was Ms Myers' comparative youth. Interventions in relation to carers are guided not only by the age of the cared-for person, but also that of the carer.

Not surprisingly given the roots of their work in counselling and psychotherapy, social workers were more aware of potential conflicts between carers and cared-for than were other practitioners. Discussing and negotiating these was regarded as a central part of their work. The more open recognition of potential conflict of interest arose in part because the more difficult cases involving interpersonal conflict or the transition to institutional care were passed to social workers; in the four cases in the study where there had been long-term social work contact, three involved complex and sometimes hostile relations between the carer and cared-for person. Mr Cooper, for example, caring for his wife with dementia, had received long-term social work support. He had, in the view of the social worker, considerable problems of his own, and their relationship in the past had been difficult, with her displaying what the social worker described as 'morbid jealousy'. The earlier tensions in the relationship were now carried over into the caring situation. The social worker clearly saw herself as trying to balance the interest between the two of them. She said she was not working towards a separation as she felt that Mrs Cooper did not want that: 'That's very important. She's the client and she does not want to be away.'

The social worker encouraged Mrs Cooper to accept respite in order to keep Mr Cooper going. However, she said that if he were being cruel to her or making her life miserable, 'Then I would have no compunction about splitting them up,' an unusually direct comment for a social worker.

The Bright case illustrates the difficult path that social workers have to tread in balancing the interests of carer and cared-for when relations have reached crisis point. Mr and Mrs Bright lived with his mother. The social worker had been involved informally with Mrs Bright senior for seven years through the day centre where she had always been a somewhat disruptive presence. The social worker spent much time talking to both sides, though this angered Mrs Bright senior who said: 'She comes here for me not you.' After various incidents, including bouts of possibly deliberate incontinence, Mrs Bright junior had reached the end of her tether, and rang the social worker repeatedly to say she would leave the house whether her husband came or not. The assistant social worker tried to mediate: 'I felt it was a shame like, a family breaking up.' She attempted to make Mrs Bright senior see how her daughter-in-law felt. Relations declined further and the family stopped talking to Mrs Bright. The social worker accepted that the source of the problem lay in Mrs Bright's personality. Matters came to a head when the son rang and said that his wife had hit his mother. At that point the assistant social worker persuaded her to go into respite, and then sheltered housing, where shortly after she died: 'Deep down I think she died of a broken heart.' The case was a difficult and traumatic one, in which the assistant social worker managed to retain a sympathetic understanding with both sides. Mrs Bright junior lauded her intervention: 'I cannot sing her praises too highly.' She appreciated the fact that she did not criticize them and helped remove some of the guilt that they felt. At no time did she try to persuade them to continue caring against their wishes, but nor did she abandon the interests of Mrs Bright senior.

As is clear in the Bright case, social workers did not always see their role in terms of persuading carers to continue, and the greater willingness of social workers to accept the possibility of the ending of care was borne out in their comments. Supporting a carer in making that decision was regarded as appropriate. Social workers would not intervene directly to achieve that result – unless the client was actively suffering – but they would support the carer in making their choice and would not attempt to persuade them to continue. Social workers responded to the possible ending of care with greater equanimity than did other service providers like home-care organizers or district nurses. They were also more relaxed about the moral problems of supporting carers who could be seen as unvirtuous or failing to fulfil their duties. The social worker in Ms Arne's case simply accepted that although she *could* do more housework for her mother, she did not choose to do so, and this was in contrast to the critical comments of the home-care organizer.

The majority of cases in the study involved only short-term social work intervention; the social workers followed conventional models of good practice in assessing the situation, arranging services and closing the case. Some of the assistant social workers, however, expressed a fondness for remaining in touch with clients, though they were aware that such activity was not well regarded by their seniors. Purposeless visiting has been criticized by Goldberg and Warburton (1979) and others. Carers, however, rarely understood this pattern of practice. Many modelled their expectations of the social worker on their experience of the GP, and they assumed that they 'had' a social worker in the same way that they 'had' a GP. They perceived their problems as chronic ones that did not go away, and assumed that social services saw things in the same light. Case closure was mystifying to them, and experienced either as inefficiency – 'No one knows who my social worker is' – or as a minor form of rejection. This pattern of practice has important implications for carers because of the diffidence that many feel in asking for help. Case closure meant that the onus was back with them to re-refer themselves, in a context where they were unclear if they had any justification for doing so. It was this uncertainty that underlay the frequent comment that what was really wanted was someone who would pop in every so often to check that they were all right and offer help if they were not: just the kind of unfocused visiting that is criticized in the social work literature. Mrs Reeves, for example, who was caring for a husband with a bad back, was very reluctant to approach social services, but commented rather wistfully: 'There must be lots of people like me that would rather struggle on if you like, rather than keep going and asking for things. And if there were somebody that would come round . . .'

Despite the wish to assess for need rather than services, it was clear that social workers were largely involved in the latter. We had no evidence of social workers going beyond standard services to negotiate complex packages. This was partly a consequence of the limited range of services available. For example, in Area I the assistant social worker involved in supporting Ms MacAllen who cared for her mother with dementia wanted to provide a sitter, but the local youth employment scheme providing this had collapsed in the wake of the changes in funding. There was a Crossroads scheme in the area, but social workers had been informed it was full and told to stop referring. Area II had no Crossroads scheme. What was available could also be very patchy. This was particularly true in Area II where there were some innovative schemes, but only operating in certain parts of the borough.

The lack of complex packages also reflected conventional habits of practice. Arranging flexible packages of care involves imagination and effort, particularly if they are to be sustained over time. It appeared that social workers would sometimes pull the stops out for a particular carer, but that they could only do so temporarily, and usually in response to some special event. Thus they *could* arrange for the cared-for person to be looked after at a residential home in the period between the closing of the day centre and the arrival of the carer, but this could only effectively be done on a one-off basis. The issue has obvious relevance for employment, and it is only by such extensions that full-time work becomes possible. In practice providing such support on a regular and secure basis rarely appeared possible. Problems also arise over limited resources. Ms MacAllen, for example, suffered misery at bank holidays through the closure of the day centre over four, and occasionally five, days. When this was put to the assistant social worker in the interview, she replied that she could perhaps arrange for the mother to go to the day hospital which was open for the extra days. Something *could* be done if she was made sufficiently aware of the problem and put her mind to it. The difficulty was that though the social worker could do something for one carer, she certainly could not do it for all. Another assistant social worker expressed the need to husband his credit in relation to services like day care, commenting that he could push through an extra allocation on occasion, but not as a regular thing.

In conclusion, social workers, like other front-line workers, do not case-seek. They deal with the potential pressure of demand by limiting their response to those cases that come to their notice. Once within the orbit of a social worker, carers are more likely to be recognized as such than is the case with some other practitioners, though recognition may not necessarily result in services. Social workers do not appear to have very clear target models guiding or prioritizing their response to carers; rather they apply a general social work approach rooted in the traditions of the profession, though for those who were untrained – the majority – the professional culture is weak and their reaction to carers more limited and routinized. Social workers do not focus their resources solely on those carers who are in crisis, although they respond to crises that became known to them. Beyond this, their responses are determined by the limited range of services available and by informal rationing procedures that mean that complex or flexible approaches are only available on a special basis.

Home-care organizers

The home-care service is the bedrock of community care both by virtue of its coverage and cost. Traditionally, it has concentrated on providing housework to a large number of people. Over the last decade there have been attempts to move away from this pattern, and home helps have been encouraged to provide personal care as well as – and increasingly instead of – housework. This has been accompanied by attempts to move from a thin-spread service, where the majority of allocations are for two hours, to a thick-spread one, where coverage is at a higher intensity. The change in title from home help to home-care service exemplifying these moves has occurred widely: change in practice has proved less easy to achieve (Dexter and Herbert 1983; Audit Commission 1986; SSI 1987a, 1987b, 1988; Sinclair *et al.* 1990).

Supporting carers has not traditionally been one of the aims of the home-care service, though this is changing, at least at the level of official policy. In the study, home-care organizers did not incorporate carers overtly into their practice. However, because they so often dealt with older couples, they tended to focus at the level of the household, with little distinction being made between the carer and the disabled person. Help was provided to the household in general, and the situation was not seen in terms of supporting a carer. Carers were thus incorporated, but as joint clients of the service. Beyond this, the predominant response was one of regarding the carer as a form of *resource*. Organizers made assumptions about the help given by relatives, and responded only where there was a clear shortfall. In the majority of cases this resulted where carers were themselves physically frail and unable to do the housework.

Occasionally organizers were faced with a shortfall in the form of the carer 'failing' to do domestic tasks. In these cases, organizers tended to be 'realists' in that they responded to the situation as it was, rather than how they felt it should be. They might criticize the attitude of the carer, and only respond reluctantly, but they still did. One model they never used was that of the superseded carer. When asked if they would ever assist a carer in giving up, they replied in terms of redoubling their support: 'I didn't tell her to give up when it was too much for her. I just increased our help.' One organizer did, however, add a personal comment, in line with the West study of lay attitudes (West *et al.* 1984) that she felt that when people were mentally 'gone', it might be best for all if they went into an institution, but she would do nothing to encourage this. Home-help organizers were more reluctant to become involved in a decision to give up caring than were other service providers, feeling that it was beyond their competence.

The issue of ending care raises the question of whether organizers ever operated on a *compensation* basis. By this we mean the provision of help in order to lighten the load of a carer who is otherwise able to perform household tasks. Earlier work by Levin and her colleagues suggested that the home-help service could be effective in performing such a role for supporters of people with dementia (Levin *et al.* 1989). There was evidence in our study that organizers did *on occasion* operate on this basis, though in all such cases the carers were either elderly or caring for someone with dementia. In the latter cases it was only in extreme circumstances, such as that of Ms Myers who was ill and had got to the point of hitting her mother, that the offer was made – although significantly in that case by a social worker.

For home-care organizers, the most important source of implicit policy was the shared culture of the office. They received few explicit guidelines on how they should respond to cases, and organizers learnt what the job entailed and how to do it largely from their colleagues. They compared cases and swapped advice. Many of the organizers had themselves been home helps; much of their practice in relation to carers drew on their own assumptive worlds regarding kinship and family life. The organizers were mostly married women in middle age, locals and largely untrained. They were more open in expressing their personal views, including ones of a judgmental or moral character, than professionals, but they were less confident about using them in their practice. Their responses were more routinized, and the scope of their discretion limited.

Despite the well-documented bias in the home-help service towards individuals living alone (who were omitted from our study), we had almost no examples of a *straightforward* shortfall of provision, at least in regard to household tasks. All carers in the study either managed the housework, received help, or had been offered help but in some sense did not want it. We shall return to this last point below. It is worth noting, however, that both areas included in the study were relatively well resourced in terms of home care (Warburton 1988); it is likely that in other less-generously provided areas or in subsequent years the shortfall would have been higher. Significantly, the only cases where a carer would have *liked* help with domestic tasks but did not receive it arose on the *compensation* basis. In all cases, this related to younger men caring for older parents, and no younger female carers expressed such a wish.

Other studies have suggested that the home-help service has been allocated on a gender-biased basis, though the extent of this has been disputed (Davies and Bebbington 1983; Wright 1986; Arber *et al.* 1988; Parker 1992). As important as the sex of the carer in this is her marital status, with a married woman sharing a household with a disabled person least likely to receive home help support (Arber *et al.* 1988). Our study was confined to people who shared a household with the cared-for person; the important distinction here was between attitudes to younger female as opposed to male carers, and to carers who were spouses.

It was in relation to the first group that the evidence of gender bias was clearest. In both areas, respondents referred to a time when there had been explicit rules and practices that discriminated against younger female relatives. Although these had been superseded or modified, it was not clear that they did not still have some force. In Area II, the old policy that debarred provision where there were relatives in the locality had been overruled at the level of the social services committee, and a new policy document that would specifically include the needs of carers as part of assessment was in the process of preparation. In Area I there had also been a shift in policy, but at a less formal level. The manager of the home-care service had told organizers that they should not be bound by the old rules, but must use their discretion. An organizer however, described the current situation in this way:

> 'We don't normally give service when there's a daughter at home. When there's a son at home and he's working, then we put service in. That used to be the rules, but we use our own discretion.'

She emphasized how:

> 'The rule's still there, but we use our discretion . . . If a son's working, you automatically give the service, if a daughter's there and she's working, I've got to think about it.'

This gendered pattern of response was reflected in the comment of the Director of Social Services of Area I that this Committee would not appove of providing a home help in order to allow a woman carer to go out to work, whereas in Area II the Director stated that the Chair herself worked and would not endorse such discrimination. The difference reflected in part a greater cultural conservatism in Area I, but it also reflected the more progressivist approach adopted by senior managers in Area II. The contrast between the two areas at the front-line level was more muted, with an organizer in Area II commenting that she believed that men did get more help than women but that this was changing.

When we turn to the situation of couples, the gender pattern is less clear. In Area I it was the custom always to put the wife as the client regardless of who was disabled; the service appeared to regard itself as primarily substituting for or supporting women in discharging their domestic duties. How far these gendered assumptions were carried through into allocation was less clear. We had one case of an older man caring for a wife with dementia, who was capable of housework and yet received help, but this appeared to have resulted as much from his expectations as a middle-class man of receiving help and his ability to marshal it, as from the response of the organizer.

Although we had no cases of straightforward shortfall in relation to housework, there were carers in the study who had wanted help of a different kind. The principal example of this was personal care. In line with national developments, both areas had moved towards including personal care as part of the official work of the home help, but the policy was in practice hedged around with provisos and uncertainty. In Area I for example, the manager said that home helps would 'assist to bath but not bath' but he was unclear exactly what this meant. Bathing in particular remained the classic grey area, only provided on an uncertain and often personalized basis (Twigg 1990b). No one in the study had been offered such help from the home-care service, though there were cases where the carer would have liked such help, had been in contact with the service, but had been led to believe that it was unavailable.

Carers also suffered from restrictions in relation to what the home help would do. These were partly explained in terms of insurance – avoiding high dusting or cleaning outside windows – and partly in terms of 'unnecessary tasks' like cleaning out cupboards, though these were sometimes precisely the tasks that the carer wanted help with; some carers gave up receipt as a result. Many female carers wanted help with the 'male' household tasks that their husbands had previously undertaken, and the home-help service geared to a traditional concept of female domestic labour was unable to provide this. Problems also arose through the inability of the service to come at defined times. One carer who worked night shifts and wanted someone to get his mother dressed in time for day care, found that the home-care service could not guarantee to come before the transport and decided not to take up the offer. The organizer explained: 'We couldn't be quite as specific as that. It's a flexible service.' It is important to note the service-oriented use of the word 'flexible'.

Certain carers remained invisible to the organizers. At the simplest level, organizers did not ordinarily meet them. 'Most of the time we don't,' commented one organizer and agreed that this made it hard for her to assess whether the carer was stressed or not. Their view of the situation tended to be constrained by the rather narrow, sectoral traditions of the service. Home-care organizers receive little in the way of formal training; their assessments were rooted in conventionally determined responses. By and large they assessed for service only, and they were rarely experienced in making wider judgments about need: one organizer in the study, for example, was unfamiliar with the term 'respite'. Contacts with social workers were limited, particularly where the service was organized separately, and sometimes made unproductive by feelings of inferiority. Individuals varied, and some did adopt a wider based approach that was informed by social work values, though in general their view – but also the remit imposed by the job – was a relatively narrow one, focused on tasks. There was a certain inevitability about this, in that by and large they offered a service that substituted for an inability to perform domestic tasks. But it meant in relation to carers that they were less likely to see the situation in terms of the *consequences* for one's life of being a carer rather than the tasks to be performed. This affected their capacity to recognize the restrictedness sometimes imposed on carers.

The Dixon case illustrates these issues. Mr Dixon was caring for his wife with severe arthritis. The organizer had only met his wife, and her impression of her was that she was 'quite a lonely lady' since her husband went out a lot and did not appear to give her much support. A sister called and helped with some of the housework, and Mr Dixon was not involved in this. As a result the organizer allocated the minimum of two hours a week and said she would be reluctant to give any more. She felt that he could do more for his wife and presented him as a rather selfish man; and the fact that Mrs Dixon went to day care three times a week was interpreted as evidence of his lack of support. The interviews with Mr Dixon and with the manager of the day centre, however, revealed a very different picture. Mr Dixon was in fact considerably involved in support for his wife, getting her up and dressed and helping her to bath. The home-care organizer was unaware of this because her remit was confined to housework, something that Mr Dixon did not do. It was clear from the carer interview that his day outings were an important safety valve, part of a conscious attempt to get away from the tensions of the situation. The home-care organizer, however, regarded them as a sign of neglect.

The case illustrates how service providers sometimes play down or even fail to recognize the impact of secondary restrictedness, and interpret attempts by the carer to develop elements of a separate life as a form of selfishness and a sign of being a bad carer. The interview with the day-care manager reinforced the significance of these aspects of visibility. Until the Dixons had gone on a holiday with the centre, the manager had thought that Mrs Dixon was rather sweet natured. But seeing her over time with her husband made him realize how difficult she could be. Mr Dixon did everything for her on the trip, and when at one point he went off for a couple of hours, the manager felt that he deserved it. He never complained, and the deputy manager described him as a 'supreme carer'. The contrast with the account of the home-care organizer is striking, and brings home how sectorally-defined views of the situation can constrain the ways in which the carer's needs are perceived.

Carers were also affected by the pattern of shifting, unstable allocations that arise from the personnel demands of the service. Provision in the home-care service is conventionally described in the literature in terms of the allocation of a defined number of hours. In reality provision is often unstable, and home-care organizers spend much of their time juggling with staffing. There was a clear discrepancy between how this was regarded by the organizers themselves – as a triumph of effort and personnel skills – and by the clients and carers, who complained that they never knew whether a home help was coming that week or whether sickness and holidays would result in a temporary withdrawal, sometimes unannounced. In making these decisions, priority was given to the unsupported, and this meant those without carers. Carers were thus exposed to a particularly unstable pattern of provision; they were sometimes subject to subtle pressures, as for example with one elderly spouse who, when he rang up to find out about cover for the home help who was ill, was asked 'couldn't you manage?'.

Sometimes the practice became withdrawal by default. Once again this was regarded differently by the carer and the organizer. The Scotts had been given a home help, but after two months she fell ill and the allocation petered out. Mr Scott decided not to pursue the matter, partly because he was dissatisfied over the limitations on what the home help could do, but partly because he felt the service was unreliable. The organizer, by contrast, presented his failure to come back as evidence that the home help was not needed. What was experienced by the carer as unsatisfactory, was regarded by the service provider as evidence of a successful outcome. In the absence of reassessment, organizers effectively run a default system that requires recipients to reassert their need. Such an approach makes sense in the context of the resource pressures they face and the practical difficulties of monitoring or reassessing cases systematically, but it puts the onus on carers to act, in a context where they are often uncertain about their eligibility, and diffident about putting their needs forward.

The move in the service towards a more closely targeted response has implications for carers. It is likely that, in the context of the withdrawal of service from the lighter end of disability, the current bias in allocation against those who share a house or have a relative nearby will continue and even intensify: unless that is the needs of carers are explicitly incorporated into the priorities of the service. This has happened in certain authorities, often in association with attempts to clarify and prioritize which clients should receive the service. How extensive this incorporation will be in practice remains to be seen.

In conclusion, the home-care service is important to carers because of the breadth of its coverage: more carers come into its orbit than any comparable service. It has a significant function to perform in lightening the load of certain carers, particularly those caring from someone with dementia where the home help can be an important source of company as well as of relief with housework. However, because of its pragmatic emphasis on housework and its relative isolation from wider concepts of assessment, some carers who come into its orbit, together with their problems, remain invisible to the service. Only rarely is help for the carer incorporated directly into the practice of the organizer. Most carers who receive help do so because they are themselves elderly, and because provision is focused at the level of the household. The relevance of the service to carers is also limited by restrictions on what it provides, particularly in relation to personal care or tasks outside the remit of day-to-day housework. Carers are also often exposed to a particularly unstable pattern of provision, and one in which they may have to reassert their needs.

Occupational therapists

There is a national shortage of trained occupational therapists (Scrivens 1983; Blom-Cooper 1989). As a result in many areas, including one of the two in the study, unqualified staff, with such titles as domiciliary occupations or rehabilitation officers, perform the tasks of an occupational therapist. (In the account that follows we will use the title of occupational therapist to cover both trained and untrained practitioners.) The employment of qualified and unqualified staff has implications for waiting lists and for the thoroughness and scope of assessments. Although occupational therapists are employed by both health and social services, in our study only those employed by social services were directly in contact with carers in the sample.

In general occupational therapists are concerned with providing practical help for disabled people. Their professional ideology encompasses a wide approach, in which rehabilitation, and functional and social adaptation in the broadest senses are seen as important, and in which the context of the client's life, including family life, is emphasized. But the realities of practice impose a narrower approach. The primary way the service helps carers is by increasing the independence of the cared-for person, usually through the supply of aids or adaptations, though some aids help carers more directly, by enabling them to perform their caring tasks with greater ease.

Unlike other practitioners, occupational therapists visit the home and see the client in his or her domestic circumstances. They were thus more likely to be aware of the presence of a carer, and had in many cases in the study met him or her, something they were explicitly encouraged to do in the policy documents of Area II. Major adaptations to the house also inevitably involve tripartite negotiations, and these once again bring the occupational therapist into direct contact with the carer. Despite this, the primary focus of their practice remained on the disabled person, and the carer tended to be described as a 'relative' or 'family' rather than as a carer as such. Occupational therapists did sometimes incorporate carers more directly such as when they provided aids that enabled carers to perform their functions more effectively. This led them in some degree to categorize the carer as a *co-worker* – an extension of the support available to the disabled person. No occupational therapists articulated a view that transcended this instrumental focus and incorporated carers' interests *per se*.

Scrivens proposes three models in describing the implicit rationing systems operated by occupational therapists working in the local authority sector (Scrivens 1983). Primary rationing, the most direct form, applies when the budget has run out and some clients will as a result receive no service. Secondary rationing is where rationing is achieved through delay and the building up of waiting lists. Tertiary rationing is where all clients receive a service, but the quality and quantity is diluted. Area II operated a two-tier system whereby cases were prioritized. The waiting time for non-priority cases was six months, a clear example of secondary rationing whereby the existence of need was diagnosed, but provision deferred. Area I did not operate a two-tier system. There was no priority category, and the waiting list was in the region of six to eight months, until the authority initiated a policy change. At that point, occupational therapists were instructed to meet only 'referred need' and not to undertake a full assessment. This reduced the waiting list to four weeks. This is an example of tertiary rationing whereby the quality and quantity of the service was diluted. Although carers will suffer under all three forms, tertiary rationing has perhaps the greater implications for them. Work with carers is marginal to occupational therapy, and is easily displaced by other priorities. Diluting the quality of the service by pushing more referrals through the system is likely to result in the carer's needs becoming invisible. This has implications for some carers of adults with physical disabilities who often have limited contact with service provision, so that if service providers like occupational therapists fail to pick up their needs, there are few alternative pathways that will lead to their recognition.

One of the consequences of long waiting lists was that carers bought their own aids or made alterations themselves. One carer asked for bath aids after her husband became stuck in the bath, but she was told she would have to wait at least six months:

> 'Of course we couldn't wait six months because Tim couldn't get out of the bath. That night he was in for half an hour. The water was freezing . . . I knew I had to buy them right away.'

Lack of choice in the supply of aids and adaptations as we have seen in Chapter 3 was identified as a problem by both carers and disabled people. The issue was recognized by service providers and managers, although they tended to see the provision of standard aids and adaptations as reasonable, given resource constraints. They varied in how sympathetic they were on the issue. One manager commented:

> 'We are providing for functional needs of the individual, not to match the decor of the house . . . We are not Littlewoods.'

Lack of choice prompted some people to buy their own aids and adaptations. Occupational therapists were uneasy about this because it meant that aids and adaptations were being provided without a proper assessment, resulting in inappropriate or even damaging equipment being used. It also meant that people remained unaware of the full range available.

Occupational therapists have to rely on other local authority departments, notably the store and the architects and building department to carry through their assessments. Clients and carers had often had to wait for an assessment, and once this was done they expected action to follow. They had no understanding of the process of supplying aids and adaptations, and when long delays occurred, became impatient, feeling they were receiving a poor service. Such delays, however, were expected by the occupational therapists who had become inured to the slowness of the system. They knew that something would eventually be done, and they had adjusted their concept of a 'reasonable' delay in line with their experience. But they did not always convey these facts to the carer. The two sides worked to a different set of expectations, causing misunderstanding and frustration.

Conflicts of interest can arise in relation to occupational therapy if the client refuses help that might assist the carer. According to the occupational therapists this was rare; the main reason for refusing help was where clients did not wish to admit their disability and its related stigma. Occupational therapists described how they sometimes had to negotiate with clients and carers in order to get them to accept adaptations to their property since many were reluctant, sometimes resulting from their unattractive nature. Problems could arise where the disabled person lived in a house owned by the carer, who might refuse to have the house adapted. Carers who lived in local authority housing were also anxious that a house, once adapted, would classify as disabled housing, and that they might lose their chance to gain under the right to buy legislation.

Although the professional traditions of occupational therapists encompass a concern with the wider social circumstances of the client, the realities of their day-to-day work, in the context of waiting lists and backlogs, mean that practice is much more narrowly focused. The use of untrained staff reinforces this. Carers may come into the orbit of an occupational therapist by virtue of the domestic location of their work, but they tend to be incorporated into their practice to only a limited degree.

Chapter 5 *THE HEALTH SECTOR*

Some of the most important sources of help for carers are located within the health sector. Three service providers were of particular significance: general practitioners, hospital consultants and community nurses. Once again the chapter refers predominantly to the situations of carers of physically disabled and elderly people.

General practitioners

General practitioners are the one service provider with whom the great majority of the population is in contact (Johnson and Cross 1983), and they are, thus, of considerable potential significance in the recognition of the needs of carers and the mobilization of help for them (Hunter *et al.* 1988). Indeed for many carers, especially those looking after someone with a chronic illness or physical disability, the GP is their only service contact; he or she assumes particular significance as a result. GPs are important gatekeepers to services. Recent policy discussions have attempted to assign them a more defined role in the new community care; the possibility of their taking overall care-management and budgetary responsibility for the community care of patients has at times been raised (Glennerster and Matsaganis 1991).

Although GPs are located at the boundary of the health and social care systems, the sources of their practice – their 'implicit policy' – are primarily medical. Unlike other service providers such as social workers and home-help organizers, formal policy is largely irrelevant to their work. GPs, although part of a network of service responses that make up community care, operate in a policy vacuum. As independent contractors of professional status, they have not been subject to line management or to the policy direction of the health authority or Family Health Services Authority (FHSA). They have discretion in how they choose to practice, and exercise considerable autonomy in defining their areas of 'competence', 'responsibility' and 'action' (Crombie 1984; Richman 1987). The main source of practice models for GPs is their professional training and culture. This defines the nature of their work and provides the intellectual and ideological underpinning for it. The approach is an essentially biomedical one in which social factors although recognized are marginalized (Huntingdon 1981). GPs have traditionally received little training in these areas, although with the new training there have been some signs of change.

Since their professional role and ideology did little to prepare them for work with carers, assumptive worlds assumed greater importance. The limits of their medical knowledge when dealing with social issues meant that GPs drew heavily on their own life experience and values. These were constructed in terms of a 'common sense' framework that was applied, in the absence of any other, to the situation of carers. GPs were less self-conscious about deploying their own assumptive worlds than were other practitioners. Their training encouraged self-confidence, and they often presented value judgments as 'objective knowledge', making them appear more absolute than actually they were. This supports Friedson's view that doctors were not always aware of the kinds of decisions that could be helped by their medical knowledge and those that could not (Friedson 1970). When making judgments about the social world, GPs employ techniques adopted from their medical knowledge. Consequently their pronouncements are often definite and absolute and do not reflect the ambiguities and inconsistencies of the social world. In comparison to other service providers, such as social workers, who stressed the importance of consultation and negotiation between the various actors, GPs were more likely to be directive in the advice they gave a carer. As one GP commented:

> 'You can't rely on carers to make up their own mind to give up caring . . . A lot of carers would carry on until they are in a worse state than whoever they are caring for, so I'd you know, I'd just tell them that.'

Carers, swayed by the professional status of GPs, often took these value judgments more seriously than if they were made by another service provider.

Although GPs acknowledged that their role was broader than the traditional medical orientation and that they had to deal with social issues in their everyday practice, most still maintained a strongly medical identity in their approach. Their primary focus was on the patient, and carers tended to be marginalized. Helping carers was not a central aspect of the GP's work, and their conceptualization of them was often vague. In so far as they did perceive them as carers, it was with an instrumental emphasis, regarding them as a form of resource.

Beyond this, GPs adopted three broad approaches to their work with carers. First there were those who had a clear carer orientation and who attempted to incorporate carers in a systematic fashion. These were in the minority and were usually younger GPs in group practices. Although responsive to social aspects, they maintained a distinction between the medical and the social role. They were generally clear when they could not help the carer, as for example with benefit advice, but did not leave the situation there but referred on to other service personnel. Second, there were those who were vaguely aware of carer issues and embarrassed they were not doing more. Their response to carers was more *ad hoc* and arbitrary. Carers had to be in the right place at the right time to receive help. The majority of GPs interviewed belonged to this group, which was the most ambivalent, contradictory and complex of the three. It was a response that reflected the broad and ill-defined nature of general practice which often gave rise to insecurity and uncertainty over the GP's role, and this in itself prevented a systematic response. Third, there were those for whom the issue of informal care was largely irrelevant, as carers had no place in their frame of reference. Carers here were not incorporated at all; they were unlikely to get help from these GPs unless as a direct by-product of the medical treatment of the cared-for person. These practitioners did not feel they were failing in their responsibilities to carers because they did not perceive that they had any.

The ways in which GPs practice can have consequences for carers which are visible and the degree to which those that are incorporated into their work. GPs typically see patients individually, for brief periods, and within the confines of the consulting room. Many carers remain literally invisible to the doctor because they do not attend the surgery or because the cared-for person goes alone into the consulting room. This is particularly characteristic of patients who are mobile and *compos mentis*. It is often only by chance that the GP discovers the implications of the situation. As one GP remarked:

> 'Even now I go into a house and I see a situation where I think "My God", you know, this person has been caring for years and you didn't even know about it.'

The degree to which the carer's situation is 'visible' can also be affected by the GPs view of the patient. One GP, for example, dismissed a patient's complaints as hypochondria, and as a result played down the implications for the carer, making the very real problems she experienced effectively invisible.

Despite the fact that they remain in long-term formal contact with the patient or carer through the system of registration, GPs provide a 'one-off' rather than 'continuing' service. They operate an essentially reactive model: each consultation forming a discrete episode, and the onus is on the patient or carer to put themselves forward if further help is wanted. The GP, of course, remains the person's doctor, but he or she does not take on a monitoring role, identifying changes in a carer's situation, but leaves it to the patient/carer to make contact. 'Continuing' services by contrast, as well shall see, remain in touch, and this fact allows them to monitor changes in the circumstances of the carer and identify new difficulties as they emerge. This can be important since carers were often uncertain as to what was appropriate support, and relied on other people to define it for them. Those GPs who, at least by the carer's account, dropped by from time to time to ask how they were, were much valued.

The way in which the needs of the carer are, or rather are not, incorporated is also affected by the nature of doctor–patient interactions. The doctor–patient relationship can be expressed as a continuum, ranging from being doctor-centred to patient-centred (Byrne and Long 1976). Doctor-centred interactions predominate. These are essentially information-gathering consultations with little attempt at open dialogue, and deny the opportunity for expression of feelings. Carers often present problems that are diffuse and want to use the consultation to talk generally about their situation. A doctor-centred consultation afforded the carer little space to do this. In accordance with their professional training, GPs liked to establish 'facts' and were uneasy about making sense of information sources that were unreliable, multiple or conflicting. The problems presented by carers, however, tended to be of this sort. Most were located in the social rather than the medical sphere, and could not be reduced to single, reliable 'facts'. This meant that the carer's experience was either reformulated within a medical definition, or overlooked since the GP did not know how to respond.

This pattern of exclusion was reinforced by the pressures of resources and time. The more holistic aspects of the GP's role are narrowed by the reality of practice, and GPs gave prominence to the medical aspects of their work. This was partly a question of pragmatics and pressure of resources, but it also allowed the GP to place clear boundaries around his or her involvement. One GP expressed the dilemma faced by many doctors:

> 'It's [informal care] just one more area to cover. I mean in general practice we have hundreds of areas and we're always left with the feeling that there are, from every consultation, from every encounter, there are another ten things we could have done . . . You know the load of carers is just another one of the 101 things which there's never enough time to do fully . . . But you know there are many things to squeeze into the time.'

General practitioners varied in the degree to which they saw giving information to the carer about the condition and its likely course as important. Some carers reported that the GP was helpful and felt supported by his or her advice and information. Some, however, felt left in the dark, and this appeared particularly the case in relation to senile dementia and schizophrenia. This echoes the finding of Levin and her colleagues in their study of dementia where two-fifths of the supporters had had no explanation from the doctor as to what was wrong with their relative. The lack of information given about the condition partly related to pressure of time, but it seemed to arise also from the emotional reluctance of some medical practitioners to address directly the needs of people who were not going to get well. Neither dementia or schizophrenia have optimistic prognoses, and GPs sometimes seemed reluctant to discuss these with carers. It is, of course, not always easy to predict the exact course of an illness like dementia; this difficulty is compounded in the case of conditions like multiple sclerosis that are fluctuating by nature. GPs in this context sometimes express concern lest they provide information too soon, in advance of the situation to be coped with or in a way that might distress or depress the carer. Carers in general valued knowing more about the condition and its likely course; it enabled them to come to terms with the situation and to adjust their expectations of the cared-for person. The latter point is particularly relevant to conditions like dementia and schizophrenia where the cared-for person is not responsible for his or her behaviour but where the behaviour can be disturbing or hurtful unless recognised as part of the illness.

Information giving was sometimes made more difficult by the issue of confidentiality. We have already noted the tendency of medicine to focus narrowly on the patient and as a result marginalize the carer. This is reinforced by the tradition of medical ethics that emphasizes the confidentiality of the doctor–patient relationship. Mr Bowd, for example, looked after his wife with multiple sclerosis and wanted to find out more about her condition, but the doctor refused to discuss it with him, saying it was a matter solely between him and his patient. Other GPs took a more flexible view and were willing to involve the carer. One commented: 'I certainly don't hold by the fact that everything's confidential and they [carers] shouldn't know anything. I think that's quite ridiculous.'

We have noted the ways in which doctors drew on their assumptive worlds in dealing with the social aspects of their work. At times GPs appeared to be operating what can be described as a moral view of caring. Several GPs, for example, expressed notions of 'virtuous' and 'heroic' carers. Although they were sympathetic to the position of these carers, they felt there was little they could do for them; ironically, that sympathy sometimes became a barrier preventing them from identifying ways in which the carer could be helped. Mrs Gorst, for example, who was caring for a husband with severe respiratory problems, was very much an engulfed carer (see Chapter 9) who had made her life around her husband and was riven with anxiety about his condition. The GP, however, was so conscious of her as a loving and supportive wife – which she was – that he failed to see that there were ways in which what he saw as her tragic situation, could be alleviated.

As part of this moral view of caring, GPs sometimes had expectations about who should help the patient and what these helpers should do. Women in particular were seen as being better able to cope with caring. As one GP commented:

> 'It may seem very sexist but certainly women seem to be much more involved with the intimate messy jobs . . . You don't really tend to expect a sort of, man to go and do a lot of intimate things, you know, or involving a lot of urine, faeces, that sort of thing, which you might expect a woman to do. You just don't really . . . You're always surprised when the men do it.'

Care by female spouses was particularly endorsed by some GPs. Commenting on the situation of Mrs Chilton who was looking after her husband with senile dementia, one GP said:

> 'Mrs Chilton is not only a carer, she is also a wife and she looks upon her role as that . . . I mean if a carer is a distant relative or a neighbour or something, then you wouldn't expect them to do the same things as you would expect the wife to do . . . Mrs Chilton being a wife can do much more intimate things than even a professional nurse can do.'

As with other service providers, GPs felt less able or inclined to intervene in spouse relationships, seeing these as a natural area of privacy. We shall return to some of the assumptions that underlie this response in Chapter 9.

Patterns of referral could also have implications for carers. The reluctance of doctors to refer to social services has been established in other work (Mechanic 1971; Ellard 1974; Bourne and Lewis 1977; Huntingdon 1981). General practitioners in the study were often ignorant about local services and few had any systematic means of finding out about them. Links with social service departments were poor, and contact with the voluntary sector patchy. Carers, however, trusted GPs to be knowledgable, and assumed that if they had not been told about some form of support or service, it did not exist. GPs were also reluctant to refer to services over which they had no direct control, such as social services and the voluntary sector, preferring to refer within the health sector. This could pose difficulties for carers whose needs tend to be primarily in the social rather than health sphere.

In conclusion, GPs are of central importance to many carers, their first port of call for help. The medical focus of their work, however, means that carers tend to be marginalized; the ways GPs practise, in a consulting room and under pressure, mean that carers often remain invisible to them. GPs have until recently received little in the way of training in the social aspects of their work, and their responses to carers were often idiosyncratic, drawing on their own assumptive worlds.

Hospital consultants

Hospital consultants are not normally included in discussions of community care. They are not based in the community, and the specialist nature of their work means that their remit is quite closely confined to the hospital and to medical activities. Their practice, however, has implications for community care, and with it for the lives of carers. A significant number of disabled and sick people, with conditions like rheumatism, diabetes, respiratory disease and heart problems are cared for within the acute hospital sector. Their GPs are involved, but the primary management of the condition is in the hands of a hospital specialist based in the acute sector. This is true also of the situation of many elderly patients, only a proportion of whom come under the care of a geriatrician. For the carers of these patients, hospital consultants were potentially important, at least by default. In the absence of any other service contact, whether or not the carer was visible to the consultant, whether or not his or her needs were recognized, they assumed particular significance – although it is a significance, as we shall see, of which consultants were often unaware.

The comments that follow relate to consultants in physical medicine. In none of the cases in the study was a geriatrician centrally involved. This should not imply a lack of concern among geriatricians for carer issues, but simply the variability of study samples. The role of consultant psychiatrists is discussed in Chapter 7.

As with GPs, formal policy has little meaning in the work of hospital consultants. Although health authorities set the overall level and pattern of resources, the clinical freedom enjoyed by consultants gives them considerable autonomy; in general, health authorities have not – at least in the past – formulated guidelines in relation to clinical practice and with it informal care. As with other professionals, therefore, the principal source of implicit policy was their professional role and ideology; this defined the focus and orientation of their intervention. Consultant physicians, not surprisingly, had a strongly medical orientation. The tradition of hospital medicine is one that focuses strongly on the individual patient, even on the individual disorder. Consultants did not in general see contact with carers as part of their work. One commented: 'One's main business is always with the patient . . . what I'm paid for . . . I'm not paid to take a social role.' Consultants were specialists, whose work focused on the particular condition. This they saw as the correct, as well as reasonable, application of their limited time. Carers were regarded as part of the taken-for-granted resources available in the community, part of the background to hospital work but not a concern of it; to this degree, they were not incorporated into their practice.

Carers came into the orbit of the consultant through the referral of the cared-for person to the hospital. Where the disability was a chronic or complex one this could involve contact over many years. In general, consultants only acted on carer issues when they became highly visible and were at crisis point. In these situations they responded in terms of the individual case, rather than any coherent or thought out policy on carers. One consultant, for example, said that he had arranged respite on an emergency basis when he felt it necessary, but he did not see this as playing any part in a wider community care policy.

The way hospital doctors practise means that carers often remain invisible to them. Consultations take place in the hospital, and it is almost unknown for a consultant in an acute specialism to visit the patient at home. The consultation itself focuses narrowly on the patient, and it is even rarer for carers to be present than is the case with GPs. As a result the existence or otherwise of the carer often remained unknown to the consultant, and decisions were made without recourse to their views. The carer also sometimes remained in ignorance of important facts that could affect their situation. Mrs Willis, for example, who looked after her husband with severe back problems, was unaware until it was revealed in the course of the interview that her husband was shortly to have an important but risky operation. He had excluded her from contact with the hospital, refusing to let her accompany him or tell her what was said between him and the consultant. She was distressed that she did not know more about her husband's condition, but she felt she could not approach the consultant:

> 'He [her husband] doesn't tell you a lot, you've just got to draw your own conclusions . . . If I went to see the doctor [husband's consultant] he would think there was more wrong with him than probably there is, you know. He would think the worst if I went, so I've never approached anyone to find out.'

As a result she remained invisible to the consultant, and ignorant about what the future held in store.

Often consultants before the interview simply had not thought in terms of 'carers' or 'caring'. Carers were not part of their workday world. The lack of visibility of the issue was sometimes reinforced by assumptions that their patients were not sufficiently disabled to need a 'carer'. One consultant presented a crudely polarized picture in which patients either were or were not capable of independent living:

'I do not have an enormous amount of contact with them [carers]. Many of the patients can look after themselves, many that can't are looked after in local authority homes.'

This was despite the fact that he had among his patients Mr Piper, who was partially sighted and had a speech impediment after a stroke as well as angina, and whose wife was heavily involved in his care. Her role and the impact of it on her life remained invisible to him.

Hospital discharge has been identified as a time of stress and difficulty for many carers, having to face radically changed circumstances, as well as new, confusing and sometimes distressing demands (Parker 1993). Consultants can play an important role at this point in mobilizing support for the carer and having regard for their needs in timing the discharge. Most were not directly involved in this way and left liaison between carers and community services to other staff such as ward sisters and hospital social workers. Such liaison arrangements, however, were not always good, and some wards had no tradition of discharge planning into which the needs of the carer could be incorporated.

Consultants regarded the issue of informal care as in the domain of other service providers such as GPs whom they saw as having a wider role that incorporated the social dimension. This view was largely shared by carers, who rarely approached consultants for help. They saw them as having a specifically medical role that was focused on the cared-for person, not themselves. Moreover, the professional status and position of the consultant often made them inaccessible to the carer and many were nervous of approaching them. To this degree carers and consultants shared the same framework of expectations. Consultants primarily mattered to carers as a source of effective medical care for the person they looked after. Accounts of the medical problems and treatment of the cared-for person featured extensively in the narratives of carers, often crowding out comments on their own situation. Securing the best possible medical treatment for their relative was something that concerned carers considerably.

In conclusion, the key to understanding the significance of consultants in relation to carers lies in the unintended consequences of their position. It is not that consultants are failing in their responsibilities to carers, but that they do not perceive themselves as having any. Their role is focused and specialized; they have, and claim, no expertise in social support. Problems arise for carers, however, when their sole contact is with a consultant, as can be the case with certain physical conditions. Here carers are linked into a service that is not attuned to their needs and may indeed remain unaware of their existence.

Community nurses

A number of writers have commented on the potential significance of the community nursing service in the support of carers (Robinson 1985; Nolan and Grant 1989; Atkinson 1992; Atkinson and McHaffie 1992a,b), and nurses are clearly relevant to many problems that carers face. This section will largely be concerned with the work of district nurses and the auxiliaries that work under them. The remit of the health visitor has always been wider than that of the district nurse, encompassing social aspects (Dingwall 1977, 1988; Robinson 1985), and work with carers thus potentially falls within their scope. In practice, however, the service has remained largely concerned with the under fives (Lucker 1979; Dunnell and Dobbs 1982); although there has been talk of a new role in relation to older people and their carers, this has largely remained unrealized (Goodwin 1988), and only one person in the study was in contact with a health visitor. The work of Community Psychiatric Nurses (CPNs) is included here in so far as they were involved in supporting carers of older people mostly with dementia. The work of CPNs in relation to younger people with mental health problems is discussed in Chapter 7.

The most significant source of implicit policy in relation to carers was the professional training of nurses; the interviews endorsed the significance of the shifts in emphasis within nursing towards a more holistic approach that have taken place over the last two decades and that are exemplified in the nursing process. The new training was seen as encouraging a wider view that extended to recognizing the needs of carers. As one nurse manager commented, the nurse now 'looks at the family unit', and this emphasis was seen as particularly characteristic of community as opposed to hospital-based nursing. There was little evidence, however, of formal policy being set by nurse managers. When asked about priorities in relation to carers or generally, a nurse manager replied that she left that to the decision of the front-line sisters, who would discuss things with her if they were unable to cope. Implicit policy, in so far as it is transmitted downwards, was through professional interchanges and day-to-day advice rather than direct policy statements.

More important than managers in determining the practice of district nurses were GPs. Despite the rhetoric of independence and of a parallel professionalism, district nurses still in large measure work to GPs. In regard to their practice with carers, as opposed to work of a more clearly medical nature, it was less a question of the GP determining the character of their work than of whether or not the GP made the initial referral into their practice. As one nurse commented: 'We don't get 90 per cent of the carers . . . if the GPs don't refer them, we don't know they are there.' It was almost exclusively through the referral of the GP or the hospital that carers came into the orbit of the community nursing service.

In common with other practitioners, community nurses drew on their own experiences of family life when dealing with issues around caring. Their comments were more overlaid with professionalism than was the case with the home-care organizers, but the references to common sense values and other aspects of assumptive worlds were still present.

The tasks that nurses perform for carers fall under three broad headings. The first concerns tasks of a clearly medical character, such as giving injections and changing dressings, that involve trained input, and where the nurses' focus is straightforwardly on the cared-for person, although their input may also ease the carer. Help with incontinence comes into this technical/medical category, though as we shall see it was not always seen in these terms, and was sometimes regarded as an optional extra.

The second group of tasks are less clearly defined as medical, and they relate to the disputed subject of personal care, the classic grey area of community nursing. Here the appropriateness of the involvement of nurses is less clear-cut. Personal care falls on the boundary between tasks of a clearly nursing character that are commonly regarded as requiring a trained nurse and the simpler tasks of home nursing that lay people are accustomed to undertake. Personal care, however, involves nakedness, touching, contact with excreta, and as such borders on areas of taboo or social constraint (Ungerson 1983; Twigg 1990b).

The third broad group of activities is more varied, and encompasses less directly task-oriented aspects of nurses' work. Community nurses have a role in counselling the carer and in giving information. All the nurses and nurse managers accepted that this was an appropriate activity, though one that was time consuming and, falling as it does under general – and unquantified – support and advice, an activity that was under threat with the move towards more time-oriented forms of audit. Nurses were also involved in making referrals, and their gatekeeping role was strongly endorsed in the interviews. One nurse manager spoke lyrically on the subject: 'they are not just the gate – they open the door – they put the key in the door and open it . . . [they are] the artery to all other services.' Nurses also had an important role to play in negotiating the situation with carers. A CPN encouraged Mrs Crowe, looking after a husband with brain damage and with behavioural problems, to develop more of a life for herself, taking up bowls and other activities.

This process of negotiation could also relate to service support; it took six months for the nurse to persuade Mr Banks to accept day care for his wife with dementia. In general nurses accepted that carers had low expectations: 'I think they have low expectations of themselves when they ask for help, as if they are not good enough. And that they needed assistance to overcome feelings of guilt over accepting help.' The continuing nature of nurses' contact was in the view of many respondents central to their ability both to understand the situation of the carer and offer support of this counselling and negotiating type. It was partly a matter of calling at the home over time and being able to observe the situation, and partly a question of building up the carer's trust:

> 'Knowing they've got someone they can turn to to ask for help, and knowing that we're here and able to give help. We don't always do the help, but if you are trusted they know they can ask you and are not afraid of asking.'

How did nurses conceive of their practice in relation to carers? Nurses were familiar with the term 'carer' and used it freely in the interviews, though they tended to refer to 'relatives' or 'family' in cases where the carers were not involved in giving physical support. 'Undeserving' carers also tended to be referred to as 'family'. In general, nurses saw carers as an important form of *resource*. All the respondents emphasized how nurses needed to support carers because they were supporting the patients. As one manager commented, carers are:

'... essential. Without carers we couldn't run the community nursing service, we really couldn't... so we've got a vested interest, if you like, to keep the carer as well as possible.'

Beyond this fundamental reality of practice, nurses had five principal bases in terms of which they incorporated carers into their practice. The first was one of *amplification*. Carers needed to be trained or have knowledge transmitted to them, so that the input of the nurse who was only there for a limited time could be, as it were, amplified. One nurse manager explained the particular role of community nurses in giving guidance to the carer:

'... far more than in the hospital. In the hospital the nurses are doing it. Now... you are going in for an hour and a half, so the rest of the hours the carers have got to look after them, so they need to know what medication, what is likely to happen. They need to know what the carers are capable of and what they should and shouldn't do... so our nurses spend a lot of time with the carer.'

The second basis was that of *standing one step back* to support the carer. Nurses often saw their role as one of helping people to care for their own, and of thus supporting and maximizing the carer's input. As one nurse commented, it was not their role to go in and sort patients out: [making them look] 'pretty in a chair and off we go... we particularly don't work like that in this area. Really we are just there to encourage carers to care.' A number of nurses emphasized how caring was what the majority of carers wished to do; what they wanted from the nurse was not interference but background support. Mr Ensbury's case provides an example of this approach, whereby the community nurses called at the weekend to see to his mother who was bedridden with dementia when the private nurses he employed did not call. They saw their role in terms of a one-step-back assistance given to a carer who remained primarily in charge. Of course the approach was – like that of amplification – not unconnected with limited resources, and the nurses admitted that they would never have been able to offer Mr Ensbury the full-time cover that he needed – and got – from the paid nurses.

The third basis of practice was that of *taking over* and substituting for the carer. This approach featured largely as something to be avoided, a way of working that had been superseded by the new professionalism. The old emphasis on doing tasks was now described in terms of 'barging in and taking over' from the carer. It was seen as a wrong way of working, although one manager recognized that it could mean that carers might feel the district nurse was no longer doing her job, as indeed some carers did think. This was, needless to say, a fruitful area for disagreement between carers and nurses, and there were carers in the study, particularly in the post-operative period, whose most pressing need was precisely for someone to come in and take over the physical burden of care.

The fourth basis was that of giving the carer a boost in order to lighten their load. This was a version of the *compensation* basis sometimes used by home-care organizers. One or two cases where the carer was given help with bathing fell into this category, since the carer was able to manage but was generally stressed. Sometimes nurses said that they took over a task because they knew the particular carer found it difficult. One nurse saw her role in terms of doing the things that carers could not face in order to allow them to do other things. This approach was most often articulated in relation to bathing and the management of incontinence, particularly across generations or genders. Nurses did not endorse any rigid pattern in this, but expressed the importance of accepting that individuals were different in what they could and could not manage. As one nurse manager commented, appealing to her own assumptive worlds, some district nurses could not bear to be bathed by their sons: 'You always have to relate to human nature . . . and how you would expect to be treated.' Among the five, the predominant responses were those of amplification and one-step-back support.

As we have seen, the potential role of the community nurse in relation to carers is extensive. This poses a dilemma for staff. Their training increasingly encourages them to see working with carers as part of their practice, but limited resources mean that they can only respond in this way in a small number of cases. This dilemma is not negotiated through any overt policy or through the establishment of priorities or targets in relation to carers. The nursing service has traditionally, in common with other medically based services, found it hard to acknowledge openly that it is rationing help (Twigg 1990b). As a result, these choices are hidden, fragmented into clinical decisions made in the context of individual caseloads. Nurses resolve the tensions of the situation by operating an 'in or out' system that enables them to protect good practice. The majority of carers remain outside the orbit of the community nursing service, and thus do not receive any of the many forms of support it can give, and for which many would be eligible. The small numbers that come into its orbit – potentially – receive the full service. As one manager explained: 'Once they are actually referred they are usually on the road to everything coming together.' This bifurcation into those who remain outside the orbit and those who are inside allows nurses to protect the ideal of good practice, since within these limited boundaries they are able to operate in terms of the holistic ideal enshrined in their training.

The process that led certain carers into receiving the full service was not simply one of initial visibility or referral. In order to get help, carers needed to be incorporated into the practice of the community nursing service, and to achieve this they either had to have a focal intervention or be related to a focal institution. As we have seen, the role of the community nurse in relation to carers falls under three broad headings: medical tasks that require skilled intervention; home-nursing tasks centred around personal care; and a series of activities around advice, support, referring and negotiating. In practice, carers only receive the third form of support where there is a focal intervention of the first type. Support of the second type is most commonly provided in conjunction with the first, but is occasionally provided on its own basis. For example, Mr Plumb looking after his elderly wife with severe mental health problems, received considerable support from the CPN. She helped him to apply for attendance allowance, suggested a sitter, talked to him on many occasions about his wife's condition and his decision for them both to go into residential care. But she acknowledged in the interview that she was only able to do this because she gave Mrs Plumb an injection on a regular basis. The significance of having such a focal intervention was borne out in other cases, such as that of Mr Dilley who received considerable support from the community nurse in the form of referrals to home help, day hospital and respite, as well as encouragement and a chance to talk. But once again this resulted from the nurse calling to give his wife an insulin injection.

Having a focal intervention did not of itself guarantee a wider level of support. Nurses varied, and some chose to ignore the needs of the carer. Mrs Todd, for example, had arranged for nurses to come and give her husband an enema. When asked if the nurses had ever talked about support for her or suggested things like respite, she laughed and said: 'Oh no! Nurses? God, the nurses are not in long enough.' By the interviewer's judgment she would have benefited from help with bathing, but she was unaware that the nursing service provided this.

The second major route to support was through contact with a focal institution. This largely applied to the work of CPNs, who were in both areas linked to the day hospitals. Those carers that were in contact with the service were well supported, with a good mobilization of additional forms of help. Mrs Gilling, for example, caring for her husband with dementia received an unusually comprehensive package of care that included day respite in hospital and at weekends in a residential home, attendance at a carer support group, a sitter, rotational care, and visits and occasional phone calls from the CPN. This had been marshalled by the CPN who had originally called because the day hospital had become aware of her problems, and the CPN had continued to support Mrs Gilling as part of the outreach of the service. It is important to note that the only way in which carers of people with dementia received any support or advice from the community nursing service was if the person they looked after had some additional physical problem necessitating nursing care or if they went to a day hospital.

Some carers, however, had needs that related to the second category of tasks – those involving personal care. This type of help did not of itself represent a focal intervention, and here the pattern of allocation was much more variable. In practice the issue turned around bathing, since no one in the study received help from the nursing service with getting the cared-for person up and dressed, a service that went exclusively to people who lived alone. In neither area was the policy on bathing clear cut, and in the interviews nurses expressed the familiar ambiguities about trying to draw the line between a medical and a social bath. They felt they should certainly be involved in the first, but were ambivalent about the second. A nurse manager stated emphatically: 'We do not have bath nurses. I am going to repeat that, we do *not* have bath nurses.' In one area they had used the ploy of insisting on a GP referral to choke off 'inappropriate' referrals for bathing.

The provision of baths within the community nursing service has traditionally been biased towards those who live alone (Arber *et al.* 1988; Badger *et al.* 1989), and not surprisingly only a small number of carers in our study received help of this sort. It is instructive to explore why they did so. In Mrs Garside's case, caring for a mother with acute mental health problems, the district nurse when asked why she offered her help replied of the mother: 'Well . . . she was such a nice clean old lady.' This appeared partly to be a question of rewarding virtue and partly a perverse pattern whereby help goes to those who least need it because they are the easiest and least offensive to help. Dalley (1988) has made a similar point in relation to hospital nurses. This inverse care law, however, only applied to carers who were assertive or, as in the case of Mrs Garside, where another service provider – the visiting warden – had been so on their behalf. Another carer had eventually been successful in getting help with bathing her mother after ten years of difficulty, but this had only resulted from a crisis when her own daughter, who had formerly helped her, became pregnant. Help had had to be provided at that point, and Mrs Payne had managed to insist on its continuance. In Mrs Crowe's case, caring for her brain-damaged and doubly-incontinent husband, help with bathing in the form of a fortnightly visit did appear to have been provided on a compensation basis with the aim of lessening her quite considerable levels of stress. But she had been in touch with a focal institution in the form of the day hospital. Some carers found intermittent baths of little help. Mr Mallet had been offered help with bathing his confused wife, but provision was so unreliable and infrequent that he decided to hire someone privately. Mr Ostley caring for his doubly-incontinent wife had felt that for bathing help to be of any use it had to come 'practically every day', and he did not pursue the service once the nurse ceased to call.

Reviewing the cases of shortfall, defined either by the carers themselves or by the researchers, no single pattern of explanation emerged. In general it appeared that it was harder to get help in bathing where the carers were not themselves elderly, and this was borne out in a comment of a nurse manager when asked about priorities between carers: 'I suppose it's wrong, but I suppose the middle-aged group who are reasonably fit probably get less priority than the young [i.e. children] or the elderly.'

Work by Arber and her colleagues has suggested that gender and household/marital status affect the provision of assistance with personal care. Carers are more likely to receive help if an unmarried adult carer is caring for an elderly person of the opposite sex and less likely to receive help if the carer is a married woman sharing the household with the cared-for person (Arber *et al.* 1988). With regard to gender, all nurses asserted that it played no part in allocation, and we had no clear evidence to the contrary. We did however have some cases where help with personal care appeared to have been more readily offered to males caring for a female. In Mr Ensbury's case, for example, the nurses accepted without question that dealing with incontinence was something that he did not want to do and that they would come in to manage this for him at the weekend. The case, however, was a complex one, and the nurses were also responding to him as a dedicated son who deserved some reward. Whether the assumptions would have been the same for a daughter was not clear. If gender plays a part, it is not through conscious policies, as with the home-help service in the past, but through the nurses accepting uncritically the social assumptions that they share with many carers.

Although bathing was a scarce resource, it was one that appeared to be allocated on a slightly hit-or-miss basis. Partly this arose from the lack of clear-cut policy, but also reflected the discretionary nature of the service whereby the boundary of provision could itself be shifted, and social baths fall in or out according to the pressure on individual caseloads. As a result, carers received very different accounts as to the existence of the service and their potential eligibility to receive it.

Some carers experienced difficulties with the community nursing service through its inability to come on time, or sometimes to come at all. Nurse managers recognized that this was a problem:

> 'We cannot guarantee what time we are going in. The nurse is going to do the injections and the terminals, they might not get there till 10 o'clock, 11 o'clock in the morning. The old woman is creating war because she has been up at six. Whereas they've [carers] done it and they say, "We've done it. Why bother coming in?" Then the nurse says, "If you can manage, we won't bother."'

There were similar problems with regard to evening work:

> If they're passing your house at seven, you go to bed at seven . . . it is very difficult, we can't be everywhere . . . All these sorts of barriers which are very bad, but we can't be there at the beck and call of everybody. It's not like on a ward where you can go to a room next door and come back to you in half an hour, if you are doing that and it's twenty miles to go to the next house, you can't keep coming backwards and forwards . . . it is particularly difficult at weekends [the carers] say, "Well you might as well not bother." I'm painting a bleak picture of nursing. I'm realistic, see.'

Support for carers almost inevitably took second place to acute interventions; carers were fitted around and after those obligations had been met. Carers both gained and suffered from the fact that support to them was created out of marginal resources. We shall return to this issue in Chapter 11. Nurses, like the home help, operated an implicit withdrawal system, especially in relation to bathing, whereby provision was allowed to lapse with the illness or holidays of staff. The carer was then required to press for the resumption of the service. One manager recognized that this method of withdrawal, leaving a telephone number for the carer, was not really satisfactory: people lost the number, or did not understand what was or was not on offer. And she acknowledged that professionals used it as a means of resolving their own difficulties.

Nurses voiced some of the same moral dilemmas over supporting carers as did home-care organizers, although in general they were less worried about helping the undeserving. One nurse echoed the view of many when she described how carers ranged from those with low expectations, across those who were 'well aware' to the 'scamps who will fiddle anything'. She felt that nurses were able to distinguish between these and act accordingly, though like others she was concerned that diffident carers missed out. Nurses clearly responded to 'virtuous' carers. Mr Banks for example was seen as dedicated to the care of his wife and as a result the considerable demands that he made were accepted:

> 'He does tend to ring up an awful lot. Sometimes he just rings when he feels like it, but I've always thought, well I shan't say anything, because it's ten o'clock or half past ten at night. It's a bit much when you've worked all day, but I never really minded because he had worked so hard with Harriet.'

We had no cases where the carer was regarded as bad or neglectful. What we did have, however, were cases where there was a slight tone of disapproval at the success of the carer in obtaining help that the service provider recognized as appropriate but regarded as over the odds. Thus in the case of Mrs Gilling, though the CPN had arranged the package, the tone of her description suggested that she felt that Mrs Gilling had done better from the system than she deserved to do. In a similar vein a manager in Area II referring to articulate carers said: 'Regretfully it does happen. I would hope not but I have a feeling that it does. If they are very nasty and ask for everything, they might get it.' The use of the word 'nasty' is significant here. It suggests the tensions that service providers face when they know support is limited and that carers in order to get it have to be assertive or 'pushy'. This raises ambivalent feelings towards the recipients; service providers sometimes appeared to make a moral distinction between 'appropriate help' and 'fully-deserved help'.

Nurses like other practitioners had to operate within the context of services that are sometimes below the ideal standard. At times they hid this fact from themselves. Thus the nurse explained that Mr Banks preferred to take his wife to the day hospital by car, whereas the interview with Mr Banks made it clear that he only did this because of the uncertainty of the transport. In a similar way, the CPN played down Mrs Gilling's rejection of the first respite home that her husband had used, recounting how she as a professional had worked with Mrs Gilling on her 'feelings' about this, whereas from the interview with Mrs Gilling it was clear that she had a number of well-based criticisms to make of the facility. The CPN had to work with this quality of respite and was reluctant to face up to its deficiencies. She also played down Mrs Gilling's loneliness, representing it in the context of the high level of support that she got as somehow unreasonable: 'I think on the whole Mrs Gilling gets out of her days what she wants to get out of them.'

In general, when asked whether they would ever support a carer in giving up care, nurses replied in terms of counselling the carer and redoubling support. A number were clearly uneasy about the prospect of a carer giving up. If the conflict of interest between the two parties was extreme they preferred to pass the case over to the GP believing that 'carers and patients usually take more notice of the GP'. Nurses felt it was beyond their remit to impose a settlement:

> 'If you see the whole family is breaking up, the husband is clearing off and leaving the wife and the kids are leaving because of this person, you've got to think of the future. Again you've got to modify your opinions. We have no right to say to somebody they should stay at home or go into hospital. It's the patients and the family and we can't interfere too much. So again you get the GP involved.'

This reliance on the GP to resolve the situation was echoed in a greater readiness of doctors to step in and make decisions for the carer.

The CPN supporting Mr Plumb expressed a more mixed view. She did not believe that nurses should always be in the business of shoring up caring situations. She accepted that there were situations where it would be appropriate to encourage the ending of care, and she cited an example of a younger person with a learning disability being cared for by an elderly parent. But when she was asked if she would have felt the same had there been no independent future, she replied: 'I don't think so.'

In conclusion, nurses are aware of the needs of carers but the pressure of caseloads and the bias towards acute medical interventions mean that carers only receive their support if there is either a focal intervention or they are linked to a focal institution. By these means nurses are able to protect the ideal of good practice, and balance to some degree the competing demands of professional ideology and resource pressure.

Chapter 6 SERVICES IN A MIXED SETTING

We now turn to services provided in a range of settings and across all three service sectors: social services, health and the voluntary sector. Here our emphasis shifts from individual service providers to service settings.

Day care

Day care is provided in a range of venues and forms (Carter 1981; Twigg *et al.* 1990a; Brearley and Mandelstram 1992). The local authority and voluntary sectors are the largest providers, sometimes in purpose-built centres, but also in temporary venues like church halls or sheltered housing complexes. Provision is mainly for older people, though as was the case in both of our areas, centres are also provided for younger physically disabled people. Day care for people with dementia can be provided in specialist centres, although ordinary day centres also accept attenders who have some degree of confusion, and this was the case in both our areas. Day care can also be provided in residential homes, although criticism has been made of its quality (Fennell *et al.* 1981; Allen 1983). Within the health sector, day hospitals tend to put less emphasis – at least officially – on the support of relatives than do social services centres. Day hospitals were developed as a more efficient and effective setting for treatment and rehabilitation than that provided on in-patient wards (Brocklehurst and Tucker 1980; Fennell *et al.* 1981). Their curative and rehabilitative focus is often subverted, however, by the long-term, essentially social, needs of many patients. Among these are the needs of carers. Providing long-term, socially based support is more accepted in the psychogeriatric sector, and here the support of relatives is recognized as a major function (Gilleard *et al.* 1984; Smith and Cantley 1985). Both of our areas had day hospitals operating on this basis.

Carers came into the orbit of day-care services through referral from a key service provider. In the case of day care organized by social services, this was usually the social worker; in the case of the day hospital, the psychogeriatrician. Often these service providers effectively allocated places, but sometimes centre managers had some discretion over referrals. Where this was the case, organizational factors such as the transport round could play a part in determining allocation. Access to day care run by the voluntary sector, although partly funded by the statutory sector, was less clear-cut. In practice, social workers and consultants tended to see it as an extension of statutory provision, regarding their referrals as straight allocations.

Pathways into the orbit of the service were clearest where the cared-for person had a congenital disability and there was a direct transfer of responsibility from children's services. Where disability was gradual in onset, contact was more variable. Mr Reeves, a man in his fifties who had a very bad back and who despite the support of his wife became depressed and isolated at home, was offered a day place in an old people's home. This he turned down as too depressing, and it was only a chance meeting in the tea-room of the local hospital that led him into the orbit of more appropriate provision. Pathways were particularly uncertain where the cared-for person had a physically disabling condition and was only in contact with medical services.

Day care is provided at very different levels across the client groups. Among those caring for someone with dementia, provision was typically between three and five days a week. The majority of such carers received some day relief, and in all cases day care had at some time been offered. By contrast, among those caring for someone with a physical disability of adult onset, whether elderly or not, provision was at a much lower level, typically one day a week, occasionally two. In addition, a high proportion in this group had not been offered a day place or did not attend a centre. Among those with a congenital physical disability or learning disability, provision was very high, typically five days a week, and nearly all in this group attended a centre. The pattern can be expressed in terms of a U-shaped curve with two parameters: intensity of provision and focus of provision (Figure 2).

Figure 2 The allocation of day care

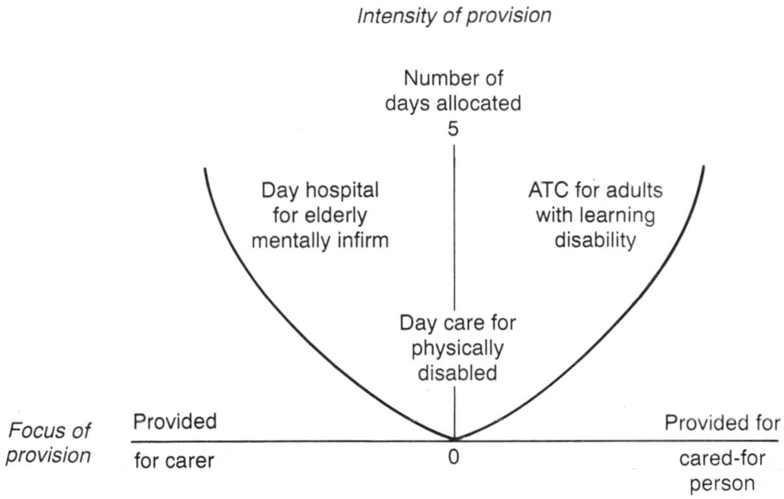

Although we discuss the situation of carers of people with learning disabilities more fully in Chapter 7, it is helpful to note at this point that these carers receive the most day-time respite, but only indirectly, as a by-product of services that aim to enhance the life of the cared-for person. The fact that the cared-for person is young and has a life before him or her is central in understanding this essentially educational model of provision with its five days a week regime. As a result, however, the carers who receive the most respite are not necessarily the most stressed, although this group does include some highly-stressed carers. Here the stress levels of individual carers are not directly incorporated into decisions about provision. At the other end of the curve we have day services for people with dementia. While these, particularly the psychogeriatric day hospitals, have not abandoned the ideal of improving the health and functioning of the cared-for person, they accept that their role is primarily one of supporting the carer. The carer's needs are incorporated into decisions concerning allocation, and provision varies according to a perception of their intensity. Provision, while not as extensive as in the educational model, can be at a relatively high level.

Between these two poles, provision is low and aims more mixed. Here day care is primarily provided for the attender, though the needs of the carer are recognized and to a limited degree incorporated into decisions about allocation. They do not, however, have the legitimacy that they do in relation to dementia. It is in this area of physical disability that conflicts of interest between the carer and the cared-for are most clearly present, and where negotiation assumes particular importance. Physically disabled people were *compos mentis* and able to express a view; and their – what we shall term in Chapter 9 'moral status' – was such that these wishes had force in the eyes of service providers. As a result they were able to refuse a place and effectively to put an embargo on this form of help to their carers. Carers, particularly spouse carers, were often loath to force the matter or to insist on their own needs in the face of the reluctance of the cared-for person. Parker (1993) in her study of spouse carers suggests that the dynamics around such service receipt may have a gendered aspect, with wives less likely than husbands to force their interests against those of their spouses.

There was ample testimony in the interviews to the benefits of day care. As Mrs Askew caring for a husband with dementia repeatedly said: 'Those two days are worth everything to me.' Strongly positive comments were most characteristic of those caring for someone with dementia or brain damage, and in a number of such cases it was hard to see, in the eyes of the researcher, how the carers could have continued without such help. Among those caring for someone with physical disabilities the need tended to be less acute and there were fewer cases where the withdrawal of the support would, again in the eyes of the researchers, have caused care collapse. This is not to say, however, that such inputs were unimportant. Mrs Reeves cared for a husband with a bad back. They were a close couple, but she was sometimes oppressed by the boredom and claustrophobia imposed on the relationship by his disability. Going to the day centre, meeting people and enjoying himself had transformed the situation, lifting his depression. The care is important because it demonstrates how even a small input – one day a week – can bring significant relief.

For day care to be helpful for the carer, it needs to be attractive to the cared-for person, and the need to attract is most significant where the carer's 'control' over the cared-for person, whether moral or physical, is weakest. This is particularly evident in relation to mental illness where the lack of good quality day occupation is striking. We will discuss the circumstances of carers of people with mental health problems more fully in Chapter 8, but it is worth noting here how few cared-for people in this group chose to attend a day centre or hospital, and that though their carers might wish for the peace of mind that attendance could bring, there was little they could do about enforcing it. The service was basically unattractive. Clients were able to exercise choice: they were mobile and the ethos of the service was not one where they could or would be coerced into going. This was in contrast to the situation of carers of elderly mentally infirm people where the carers' 'moral' and sometimes physical predominance meant that they could encourage or cajole their relative into attending. This is not to say that some of them did not experience difficulties or qualms in doing so, but these were in large measure overridden. Day care managers were also willing to be more proactive and would sometimes 'bounce' the elderly person into accepting the service.

Even where support for the carer was recognized as one of the aims of the service there was, as in other studies (Carter 1981; Smith and Cantley 1985), little in the way of structured contact with carers. Contact was *ad hoc* and infrequent, dependent on chance encounters or on the carers coming to the centre or ringing, often about transport. Carers had to make themselves visible. As a charge nurse at a day hospital for elderly mentally infirm people said: 'My involvement with the carers is minimal really. If they come in, I see them. I may never see them.' The view of day care staff appeared to be relatively narrowly circumscribed, restricted literally by the boundaries of the building. Managers and staff rarely, if ever, went to the house of the attender, whose life outside the centre remained hidden from view. Staff relied on the initial account given by the social worker or other practitioners who made the assessment, but this recorded information was often out of date and partial. One manager of a centre for older physically disabled people felt the lack of an extension arm: 'It would be good to have a social worker, where you could pick up the 'phone and say, "I'm not too happy about Mrs so and so."' As we have seen CPNs did operate in this way in relation to certain day hospitals, picking up changes in the carer's situation – in Mrs Gilling's case no longer coming to the carers' group – and being able to offer new forms of help. Thus, despite the strictures above concerning contact, day centres and particularly day hospitals were sometimes able to operate as a focal institution linking carers to other forms of help. Day care, as we shall see, operates as an important feeder mechanism into respite, and the fact that day-centre staff, potentially, have contact with the carer over time means that they are well placed to negotiate the acceptance of what can be a difficult service for many carers.

Attendance at day care sometimes made visible the difficulties that carers faced. Staff might not see the situation at home, but they did have a chance to observe the disabled person in an ordinary living setting, and got to know the problems they might pose for others better than the practitioners who had originally referred. Contact over time sometimes revealed new aspects, as the case of Mrs Dixon described in the section on home care illustrates, whereby the difficulties she posed for her husband were only apparent to the day-care staff and not to the home-care organizer.

One of the limitations of the usefulness of day care was the length of the day. Most day care effectively operates only from 10.00 a.m. to 3.00 p.m., and some carers found this frustrating. Mr Chappel who cared for his elderly mother and worked nights commented: 'I haven't a chance to turn round before she is back.' For some elderly carers who were not under great stress, the truncated day was not a problem; to an extent it reflected their own patterns of going out. But for the most highly stressed, or for those who had clear ideas about what they would like to do, the short day was frustrating. It vitiated the attempts of Ms MacAllen, a woman in her fifties looking after her mother with dementia, to meet people since the civil service club she wanted to attend was held in the afternoons. For any carer who wanted to work full time, it was useless. Although some service providers talked about the possibility of packages of care that could be linked to other forms of service in order to make a longer day, none of the carers in the study had received such help. The two day hospitals in Area II were considering seven-day opening although both envisaged problems over resources and staffing. One centre for physically disabled people in Area I was run on more recreational lines, open at the weekends and on some evenings, and this brought a welcome flexibility to carers. Closures were a source of strain for some carers, particularly those who were highly stressed and relied on the centre for relief from the behavioural problems of the person they looked after. Ms MacAllen described graphically the misery of bank holidays when she was left alone with her mother who had very severe dementia for four, sometimes five, consecutive days.

The unreliability of transport was recognized as a problem by both carers and service providers. Transport often failed to collect clients on time, leaving the carer to wait around as the cared-for person became restless, and returned them at any time between 2.45 p.m. and 4.30 p.m. This unpredictability ate into the carers' day; carers could not risk being out for the full period in case their relative was dropped off before the scheduled time. Ms MacAllen described turning the corner to see the ambulance unloading her mother on the doorstep. Sometimes the problem of transport became so dominant that assessment was for transport rather than day care. As one manager admitted rather ruefully: 'We fit them [the clients] in when it suits us.' The difficulties caused by transport have been repeatedly identified in research (Sinclair *et al.* 1990). It remains unclear how far they are solvable. Drivers have to negotiate not only local traffic conditions, but also unpredictable situations in clients' homes. There were some indications, however, that where the issue was given priority, as was the case with some services for younger congenitally disabled people or people with learning disabilities, a better and more individual service, sometimes using taxis, was provided. This, however, required extra resources; there is evidence from other studies that transport already represents up to a third of the cost of day care (Fennell *et al.* 1981).

In general, service providers felt that there was little they could do about the unreliability of transport: it was out of their control. As a result, some carers brought the cared-for person themselves. Service providers tended to play down the significance of this, emphasizing instead its benefit in the form of a chance to meet the centre staff.

Unlike some other studies (Lewis and Meredith 1988; Sinclair *et al.* 1990), we have no evidence of disabled people being 'too bad for day care' and returned to the sole charge of their carers. All the centres in the study attempted to cope with incontinence and aggressive behaviour, and where this was impossible referred to other provision. We did, however, have a case where a carer was very anxious that her husband's violent behaviour might lead to his losing his place at the centre, and she feared that she would be unable to cope were that to happen. Her fears were in fact misplaced and the centre had no such intention. For the manager and staff, Mr Askew's violent behaviour was a taken-for-granted aspect of his condition and not an issue. Mrs Askew, however, did not know this. Understandings and assumptions shared by service providers are not always shared by carers, and anxieties that are unreal to practitioners may still have to be allayed.

Day care is an important form of support for carers, particularly those looking after someone with dementia for whom it can be a lifeline. Managers and referrers recognize this fact. The degree to which the needs of the carer are overtly incorporated into their allocation decisions varies, however, according to the client group and the predominant focus of the facility.

Institutionally-based respite

Respite can be provided in local authority homes and hostels, in private residential homes and voluntary sector facilities, in designated respite units, and on acute and long-stay wards. There are also flexible, non-institutionally-based respite schemes that provide relief either in the home of the disabled person or that of someone affiliated to or employed by the scheme (Thornton and Moore 1980; Thornton 1989; Twigg *et al.* 1990a; Leat 1992). Although the two study areas contained a ranges of institutional respite facilities, there was little or no flexible provision, and we had no examples of its use in the sample. Other work, however, suggests that such provision is more likely to be acceptable to carers and meets many of the criticisms that have been laid at the door of institutional respite (Allen 1983; Oswin 1984; Wright 1986; Twigg *et al.* 1990a; Leat 1992).

In both areas there were designated respite beds, organized according to the client group status of the cared-for person. Elderly mentally-infirm people were admitted to residential homes where possible, with hospitals taking people who were more disturbed or who needed extensive nursing care. A specialist respite unit formed in the wing of an old people's home had been created in Area I to meet some of the problems that arise from the marginal use of residential resources for respite (Allen 1983; Twigg 1989b). For younger physically-disabled people, however, facilities were more limited, and often inappropriate. Area I had no specialist provision and respite had either to be provided in a residential home for elderly people, something disliked by all, or some miles outside the borough in a home run by a national charity. Area II has designated beds in a specialist residential facility. This was, however, a model of provision for disabled people that had been inherited from the past, and would not now be the choice of managers.

Respite illustrates well the distinction between a carer service and a carer allocation. Although both areas had designated respite beds, this was not the full extent of provision. Respite was also provided on a discretionary basis, most commonly in the health sector where consultants were able to use acute beds as a means of giving relief to a carer. Sometimes beds were designated to be used in a flexible way – as for example with the GP beds in small local hospital in Area I – that could encompass respite, though they were not referred to as respite beds, and it was their allocation as such, rather than a specific designation, that determined what level of support was available. Acute medical admissions were also sometimes used by consultants to give relatives a break, though this practice tended to remain hidden, as it was contrary to the policy of the health authorities.

Most carers come into the orbit of the service through referral from a service provider, usually a social worker, a GP or a hospital consultant. Access to designated hospital-based respite is often directly in the control of the consultant geriatrician or psychogeriatrician, and carers have to make their needs visible to them. One nurse commented that the provision of respite depended on how 'practical' the consultant was; nurses often had an important role to play in bringing cases to their attention. There was a particularly clear association, across the service sectors, between day care and respite: everyone who went into respite care also attended day care. This association is something that has been found in other work (Allen 1983; Levin *et al.* 1989). Furthermore, in the small number of cases where there was a clear shortfall (where the carer wanted respite but did not receive it), the cared-for person had not attended day care. The link is partly explicable in terms of the common function of the two services: carers who need institutional respite are likely to have been offered the lesser form of day respite first. But the association also operates through the role of day care as a focal institution. As we have seen, day care offers a focus for negotiation where contact is not one-off but continues over time.

Although several carers expressed gratitude for respite, few spoke warmly in its praise. This should not be seen as indicating lack of impact or importance. Respite is commonly a service of last resort, and those who receive it are among the most highly stressed. Mr Cooper illustrates the ambivalence many feel. He cared for a wife with dementia and was torn between wanting her with him and finding her behaviour unbearable. When asked if he wanted more respite, he replied angrily:

> 'No, because she's three days at day care, two weeks in the nursing home. Well she's not getting much time at home is she? She's just being pushed about like an animal. But I can't help it. If I did not get that sort of help, I would not manage. I just say I'll keep going as long as I can, and that's it.'

For many carers the experience of respite was a distressing one and many, particularly those caring for someone with dementia, were concerned about the quality of care, about run-down facilities, possible deterioration, the impact of more disturbed attenders, and the poor quality of life in some places. As Mrs Gilling said: 'They are allowed to wander, there's no individuals and long corridors and wheelchairs, and there is no company.' Ms McAllen used respite against her inclination because she knew that without it she could not continue, but she commented:

> 'Oh they are kept clean, but they are not allowed to wear their own clothes . . . because everything is pulled off at night time and thrown into a laundry bag . . . No undergarments, laddered stockings, no means to keep them up, no bras . . . the dresses they have on, the hems are hanging out, sometimes all the sleeves split open. You know it breaks my heart because I always keep her nice.'

Observing dementia *en masse* can be a distressing experience and it was not always possible for carers to disentangle this from their feelings about the quality of care. There were, however, serious quality issues raised in the interviews, and concerns about them sometimes prevent carers from taking up respite. Not all their reluctance arose from guilt.

In those cases in the sample where carers had experienced more than one form of respite, their preferences were clear, though unsurprising. They preferred the facilities that were well staffed, newly furnished and that offered a warm and homely atmosphere. They did not want their relatives wandering around decrepit buildings in torn and shabby clothing. But as Ms McAllen discovered such preferences were often of no avail. Her mother usually went for respite to the local hospital but on one occasion a junior doctor remarked that she was not really bad enough for the main wards and referred her to a new unit at a community hospital. Conditions there were much more attractive with pleasant furnishings, single bedrooms and social areas for visiting. But when she came to collect her mother, the sister took her aside, and asking where she lived, told her that the hospital was not for people in that locality and it would not be possible for her mother to return.

Which carers received respite support? The most common provision was for the carers of people with dementia; service contact among this group was extremely high. All carers of mentally infirm people in the study had either used respite (about half), or been offered it and turned it down. A number of the users in this group were spouse carers. This was in contrast to the carers of elderly physically disabled people, where no spouse had used respite, a finding echoed in Parker's study of younger spouse carers (Parker 1993). In the few cases of use, the relationship was one of sibling. A small number of spouse carers said that they would have liked respite, but that their spouse was so opposed to the idea that it had never been seriously discussed. There were other cases where the wish was not articulated but where, in the view of the researchers, the service had potential relevance. It was unclear how far this pattern of provision resulted genuinely from the wishes of spouse carers, or whether service providers were amplifying and exaggerating values held in society about marriage, and thus failing to negotiate the service actively with these carers.

Whichever was the case, it was clear that relationship was a major factor mediating the receipt of respite and we shall return to this in Chapter 9.

Young physically-disabled people were a more heterogeneous group. The only cases where spouses used respite were where the cared-for person had a form of mental impairment such as a severe stroke; there are obvious parallels here with the use of respite by spouses of people with dementia. In relation to young people with congenital physical disabilities, two out of the three carers used respite regularly. But in both of these cases the mothers saw respite care as being of long-term benefit to their daughters, although active negotiation had also been needed to persuade them to accept it originally. The importance of the benefit to the daughters was endorsed by the service providers who saw rotational care as a means of fostering independence. The joint benefit was an important factor in the acceptance of the service by both service providers and carers.

Once carers were within the network of respite, the question became one of the amount of help received. It was here that shortfalls, in the eyes of both carers and service providers, most often occurred. The pattern of provision was almost wholly service led. The amount and pattern of use were determined not by the carers but by the respite facilities. In both areas these were under pressure, and carers had to take what was offered to them. In general, this was not a great deal. Many carers received only a fortnight a year, with provision being focused on allowing the carer to have an annual holiday. Some centres, however, offered more extensive support organized on a rotational basis. Though such provision was welcomed by carers, it was clear that the patterns of use were set by the facilities rather than the carers.

One or two people did get a great deal of respite. These were typically highly-stressed carers looking after someone with dementia. It was accepted that these were situations 'on the brink'. In these cases service providers did not regard keeping the carer going at all costs as the overriding aim: they accepted that it was likely that the cared-for person would have to go into institutional care (if they did not die before that point). In offering extensive respite, they felt they were responding to the wish of the carer rather than exploiting their capacity to continue. In some cases, service providers tried to prepare the carer for an inevitable transition.

Some carers believed that service providers discriminated against younger carers. One middle-aged man caring for his mother said he had been told that the respite beds at the hospital were reserved for the support of elderly carers; he did finally get respite, but not as much as he wanted. Mr and Mrs Bright felt that they had been implicitly criticized by the staff of the residential home when they left his mother there. It is hard to determine if there was such a bias in provision. No service provider expressed such a view, though there are obvious parallels with the priorities that appear to operate in the home care and district nursing services with regard to younger carers.

In general, service providers – both referrers and managers – accepted that conflict of interest lay at the heart of respite; their concern was to minimize it. They tended to take the view that the long-term gains to the cared-for person justified the distress or deterioration that a number of studies have identified

(Kelson 1985; Rai *et al.* 1986; Wright 1986). However, they were unlikely to press the issue where the cared-for person was fully *compos mentis*. In these cases, they regarded his or her wishes an having priority in the situation. In this, service providers were reflecting a wider pattern of response in relation to the 'moral status' of the cared-for person (see Chapter 9). In the case of Mr Lloyds, however, who had brain damage, the staff at the home were willing to 'encourage' him strongly to accept the spells of respite he disliked, emphasizing how his wife was threatening to divorce him. Though they were willing to support her quite strongly in encouraging him to go, there were limits on how far they would intervene. Had the situation become any more fraught, the manager said, she would have referred the matter back to a social worker.

A small number of service providers took a different approach to respite and were less willing to accept the inherent trade-offs involved in the service. They were not the managers, but the potential referrers; they tended to be more distant from the process of respite. Thus one GP expressed doubts about ever referring elderly people for respite because he regarded any contact with the hospital environment as potentially detrimental. It was unclear if he took the same view of respite in other settings: not untypically, a hospital base was the only one that came to his mind.

Contact with the respite facility tends to be of short duration and only episodic; staff based there play only a limited role in monitoring and negotiating the situation. As a result, respite facilities did not operate as focal institutions in the way that day centres and hospitals did. The one exception was hospital respite for people with dementia, where there were close links between the ward and the day hospital, and where the consultant had overall charge. In these cases, respite was part of an integrated service.

In line with other studies, we found that some carers would have liked to use institutional respite on a more flexible and informal basis. This was, however, often in conflict with an economically rational use of resources, there being a direct trade-off between high bed occupancy and flexibility. Some carers, for example, wanted to use respite for a weekend, but in a number of residential homes, respite weeks ran from Saturday to Saturday, with the result that a bed had to be booked for two full weeks. Service providers were naturally reluctant to do this. Provision was not always so rigid. One manager when asked about flexible breaks said: 'We have done it. It is often quite difficult when you've got, generally got, people in for a week or a fortnight, but it's not impossible.' In general the message was that provision *could* be offered flexibly, but only with some difficulty. This echoes the point made earlier in relation to social work and flexible packages of care.

Last, there was the question of whether it was possible for someone to be 'too bad' for respite. We did have two cases described in an interview with a line manager where it appeared that this was the case. One cared-for person was described as being heavily overweight, and staff said that they could not cope with her, although the carer asserted that she managed. According to the manager, the case was complicated by the feeling of the staff that the daughter had her mother at home only in order to claim attendance allowance: [She] 'liked very very regular holidays . . . I mean on a monthly basis, she liked to get away and wanted us to care for this old lady, and eventually the staff said, look, sorry, we just can't cope with this woman.' We do not have full details of the case since it was only reported in an interview. It was striking, however, how the carer was labelled as over-assertive in wanting regular breaks, in the context of caring for someone who strained the resources of professionals. It appears that it is possible to be 'too bad' for respite, but no too bad to be cared for at home. The case illustrates how the rationalities of service provision – in this case what you can expect staff to cope with – can be at odds with the situations that face the carers.

Respite is a service of central significance in the support of carers. Service managers and referrers recognize that this is its primary function and incorporate carers fully into their allocations. Because of the ambivalence that many carers experience over accepting respite, it is a service that requires careful negotiation and sensitive handling. Quality issues also need to be addressed.

Carer support groups

Carer support groups are one of the few forms of support directly provided for carers. Groups are organized in a number of ways, and are found in all three service sectors (Twigg *et al.* 1990a). Some are offshoots of the facilities like a day hospital; others are free standing. Some are generic, open to all carers; others focus on a particular client group, even a particular medical condition. Some are very much for the carers; others have a shared emphasis on the carer and the cared-for person. Some are linked to national charities; others are only local. We had examples of all such forms in the two study areas.

Where groups were attached to a facility, carers came into the orbit of the service through the attendance of the cared-for person at the centre. Such groups tended to be seen as part of the outreach of the service, and service personnel often attended. Where the group was free standing there was no natural feeder mechanism; these groups sometimes experienced difficulties over recruitment. Carers are not always easy to contact, and the nature of their lives means that they are often isolated socially. Groups that provide an individual contact person who would accompany and introduce the new attender were more successful.

As with other studies, we found that carers valued groups for the mutual support that they could bring: the chance to meet people in a similar situation and share problems and experiences in an empathetic way (Glosser and Wexler 1985; Hinrichsen *et al.* 1985; Hettiaratchy and Manthorpe 1992; Toseland *et al.* 1992). Although some of the groups in the study did offer carers the chance to express powerful feelings, in general they operated at a lower emotional key. This was, as we shall see, sometimes a source of frustration for the professional involved. Groups were also important as information exchanges. Sometimes this happened in a formal way when a speaker attended to talk about some aspect of caring or service provision. This could be helpful, though one carer resented the ways speakers ran on, dominating the evening, and excluding opportunities for the carers to talk. This echoes the finding of McLachlan *et al.* (1985) that groups with a solely instructional format were unsuccessful. As important, however, was the role of the group as an informal source of information, particularly about benefits and services, a form of exchange that was valuable since many carers were not only uncertain about what was available, but also about what it was appropriate for them to ask for help with. Hearing of the success of others was encouraging, and gave legitimacy to their own requests. Groups could also be influential in enabling individuals to perceive themselves as carers, and such self-identity could be important in making them more self-assertive in seeking and accepting service support. We shall return to this question of self-identity in Chapter 9.

Where professionals were involved or where the group was associated with a facility like a day hospital or centre, it could act as a bridge between carers and key service personnel. Carers found such informal but regular contacts useful in discussing problems or letting practitioners know of changes in their circumstances. Professionals also emphasize these aspects. One social worker who organized a relative support group saw it as a cost-effective way of meeting carers, a similar point made by a day-hospital charge nurse who saw the relatives' group as his only sure route to contact. Smith and Cantley (1985) present a more sceptical account of this relationship which makes plain the ways in which such meetings can be used by staff to channel and defuse individual discontent, to relieve the medical staff of demands for individual consultations, and to present an optimistic account of the cared-for person's condition and of the hospital as an active therapeutic institution – something that is important in maintaining staff morale.

Some groups are involved in providing significant social and recreational facilities for carers. It was striking that the most successful groups in the study were those that operated on this basis, often in the evenings from a community centre and providing a large and sociable group of people. In all cases these were either parent groups or were attached to a recreational-style day centre for physically-disabled people that also operated as a community resource. Such groups were predominantly self-help, and in the control of the attenders themselves. Service providers did not always see eye to eye with them. Groups run by social workers or psychiatric nurses, usually for the carers of older people, tended to be less sociable and also less autonomous. There is a critical distinction to be drawn between groups that are organized and to some degree controlled by professionals and those that are genuinely in the hands of their members (Twigg *et al.* 1990a).

Carers and service providers sometimes differed in what they saw as the function and benefit of a group. Some professionals had an image of the group derived from a therapy model in which there was an expectation that strong feelings would be ventilated and that the group would 'work' on its problems. This was in contrast to the expectations of the carers who were largely untouched by psychotherapeutic culture and who simply looked to the group to provide company. One CPN attached to a day hospital felt that the group had become a place for 'chit chat', and she instituted changes to move it from this social orientation to a more therapeutic one:

> 'I made it clear to the old timers that if they wanted a social chit chat they would have to go elsewhere . . . If they want to strike up a friendship then I think it is their own responsibility to get on and do that . . . they should be able to strike up a friendship themselves, after the group.'

Mrs Gilling stopped coming after these changes were instituted. Differences also emerged over the issue of cliques. Professionals tended to want to break these down and assert that the group was open to all; attenders on the other hand saw them as natural patterns of socializing, and valued the real friendships these implied.

Carer support groups did not appeal to everyone, and several carers said they were not interested in hearing about other people's troubles, as they had enough of their own. One man described the local multiple sclerosis group as 'a moaning load of buggers'. Some wanted to use the few opportunities they had to get out to enjoy themselves and to forget about caring. Some, particularly where the association was organized around a disability group with a deteriorating prognosis like multiple sclerosis and where carers and cared-for both took part, found attending only made visible their own future in a depressing way. Needs also changed over time. Some carers had valued the chance initially to talk and unburden, but having been through that experience, either left or sought a different focus, one that emphasized advocacy or recreation.

One of the problems groups faced was their marginal character, and the perception of them as a low-cost solution. Setting one up was often seen as a means of 'doing something' for carers locally, but at little or no cost. They were often funded out of marginal resources and individual goodwill. One area had a stated policy to encourage support groups at day centres, but provided no resources to do so. A generic carers' group that was run by a social work team again had no allocation of funds and as a result had to meet in a large unsuitable room in the town hall, with refreshments provided from the 'flexible' use of petty cash. The social worker who organized the group was expected to do so in his/her spare time. The problem of marginal resources also affected the degree to which the groups could offer substitute care so that the carers could attend. This was particularly a problem for groups that were not attached to a facility. Transport could also be a problem. Only one group in the study was able to provide this; most carers had to find their own way or rely on lifts. In general groups were run on the goodwill of carers and service providers, and in spite of these resource constraints.

Chapter 7 *CARERS OF PEOPLE WITH LEARNING DISABILITIES*

In the previous chapters we have examined service responses to carers of physically disabled and older people. We now turn to the circumstances of people caring for an adult with a learning disability. Although caring in these circumstances shares many of the same features, in certain important respects it is different, and these differences have consequences both for the experience of caring and the response of service provision.

The experience of caring: how is it different?

'Learning disability' is a generic term covering a range of disabilities. Most are congenital, affecting a child's brain function and learning ability. The causes are varied and sometimes unknown. Carers in the study looked after people with learning disabilities such as Down's syndrome, cerebral palsy, hydrocephalus and hypercalcaemia. Many of the difficulties these carers faced are common to caring, across the caring groups. They have been described in Chapter 3. The parallels across the caring groups have been endorsed in other work (Bayley 1973; Carr 1976; Jaehnig 1979; Byrne and Cunningham 1985; Quine and Pahl 1985, 1989; Jones 1988; Hubert 1990); thus the financial impact of care, employment and housing difficulties affect carers irrespective of the cared-for person's disability. Carers of people with learning disabilities also undertake physical tending, experience restrictedness, and need someone to talk to. There are, however, differences.

The type of learning disability obviously determines what the carer does. When this is a profound mental and physical disability, caring for someone with a learning disability is similar to caring for someone with congenital disability, involving considerable amounts of physical tending. Carers described how they had to lift, wash and dress the cared-for person and deal with incontinence, feed and care for them through the day. These carers face a demanding role, and support with these tasks was much valued.

For most carers of people with learning disabilities, however, physical tending was relatively unimportant. More significant was the impact of behavioural problems, and these give a particular character to the experience of caring for someone with learning disabilities. The nature and intensity of these problems varied greatly between individuals. Even where they were not 'severe', they were still stressful. Mr Cooke, for example, described how his son was often intractable; Mrs Trolle described how her sister, who suffered from Down's syndrome, had tantrums when she could not have her own way; Mrs Parks identified her daughter's insistent talking as 'maddening'; Mrs Bradley identified her daughter's need for constant attention as the most difficult aspect of caring. Allowing the carer time away from the cared-for person eased some of these problems, and carers valued breaks offered by day care and longer term respite. These venues, however, did not always, in the carer's view, provide support in rectifying these behavioural difficulties, and indeed some regarded attendance at a centre as contributing to the problem. Mrs Trolle, for example, felt her daughter had more tantrums at home because the Adult Training Centre she attended encouraged her 'unrealistic expectations'.

The sense of 'being responsible', as we saw in Chapter 1, is a common element in all caring, but it assumes particular importance in relation to learning disabilities. It lies at the heart of restrictedness that many of these carers experienced, for often this arose less from concrete limitations than from a general anxiety about how the cared-for person might be faring in their absence. Several carers, for example, would not leave the cared-for person alone in the home for fear they answered the door or had to face some unexpected situation that they could not cope with or that was threatening. As Mr Robinson, who cared for a son with hydrocephalus and who appeared superficially competent, commented: 'It is the old story, isn't it? – You feel safe until something happens.' This generalized anxiety meant that these carers were often more restricted than it at first appeared. As we have seen in Chapter 3 this form of restrictedness is often less visible to service providers than the more concrete forms. In the case of learning disabilities, it can also be an area of direct conflict of interpretation between service providers and carers, with service providers regarding this anxiety as a symptom of overprotectiveness. These carers also ofter suffered from secondary or shared restrictedness. Some, particularly single-parent carers, had so made their lives around the needs of their offspring that they lacked any alternative focus. They often relied upon the cared-for person for company and a social life, and were thus forced to share in their limitations.

The sense of being responsible extends also into the future. As we shall see, most of these carers are parents who can expect that their offspring will outlive them by many years. Securing a safe and acceptable future for them was a major concern, and one that to some extent affected decisions in the present.

Caring and relationship

In the study sample, most people with a learning disability were cared for by a parent. This reflects national patterns (Ward 1990). The overlap between relationship and disability, however, gives rise to particular normative expectations. Parents regard caring as an extension of their earlier childcare responsibilities, and these remain powerful in structuring their expectations. They thus assume that they will remain primarily responsible for the person they look after and in control of the main decisions regarding their care. As we shall see, this is a potent area of conflict between parents and service providers. Independent living and the problems of securing a decent future for the person with the learning disability after the carer's death are central to the experience of parental carers.

The nature of service provision

There are two features of services for people with learning disabilities that mark them out from other services described in this book. First they are integrated, managed and planned predominantly according to a social care model of provision. Carers rarely mentioned medical services, and the service providers they identified were all found in the social care sector, the majority being managers of day centres/Adult Training Centres (ATCs). Second, these services operate in the context of particular philosophies, most notably those associated with normalization, independent living and self-advocacy. As a result, there is a coherence to them not found in services for older people or people with physical disabilities where provision is much more fragmented.

For these reasons, we take a slightly different approach in this chapter from the rest of the book. The section that follows explores the help and support carers receive from individual services – Adult Training Centres, overnight respite and social work – and the remaining part of the chapter examines the impact of service philosophy, tracing its consequences for carers.

Adult training centres (ATCs)

Both areas still operated ATCs, although, as we shall see, reorganization was taking place. Young people with a learning disability usually transferred from educational and child-care services to day care with little difficulty. There were, however, a small number of cases where the pathways had not been smooth. Mrs Whitcombe looked after her daughter, Rachel, who was profoundly mentally and physically disabled. For 14 years Rachel had attended a unit for people with profound disabilities, but policy changes altered the role of the unit which meant that Rachel could no longer stay. There seemed no obvious place for her. As the months went by and no decision was made, Mrs Whitcombe became increasingly anxious, fearing that *no* provision would be made and that she would be left in sole care of her profoundly disabled daughter. In fact, social services knew that they would have to provide something; it was just a question of sorting it out. But this fact was not conveyed to Mrs Whitcombe. As the manager of the unit commented:

> 'There were several times when the adult services were totally unprepared and hadn't applied themselves . . . The result is that Mrs Whitcombe had a hard, anxious time because she didn't know. If you know how social services work and you are within that little group then you can understand that probably a service would be offered, it would eventually arrive. But that doesn't help parents who have reasons for anxieties.'

Problems could also arise at the other end of the spectrum of ability. Mrs Park's daughter had fallen through the net after school, and the situation was only remedied when her general practitioner, noticing the strain Mrs Parks was under, made a referral to social services. Service providers, keen to endorse independence, were increasingly using community-based educational placements in preference to specialist ATC units. These placements could be very successful, but the looser, more fragmented nature of this provision, meant that structures for monitoring the situation were not always present. Mr and Mrs Robson and their son Tony found themselves unsupported after an alternative placement to day care failed. Tony, who had hydrocephalus, had been offered a place on an independent living course at the local college of further education but this was not successful and after six months Tony dropped out. At that point the situation was not picked up and he spent all his time at home with no outside activities or interests. The Robsons had fallen out of the orbit of services, lost to view.

As we have seen in Chapter 6, carers of people with learning disabilities received the highest level of day-time respite compared with those of other disabilities. Only three people with a learning disability did not attend a centre and of those who did attend, most went five days a week. The respite obtained by the carer, however, was indirect, a by-product of a service that aimed to enhance the life of the cared-for person. The person with the learning disability rather than the carer was the focus of provision and support for the carer was often not openly recognized as an aim of the service. Carers were seen as part of the taken-for-granted background to provision. Carers largely accepted this and mainly spoke of the benefits of day care in terms of stimulation for the person with the learning disability. None the less, many carers also spoke of the benefits they acquired, particularly in terms of relief from day-to-day responsibility for the cared-for person.

Most carers of people with learning disabilities, because of their parental responsibilities, expected to have some involvement in the cared-for person's placement. Service providers, despite the reservations outlined below, usually accepted this. As a result there was more in the way of structured contact between these carers and service practitioners than was the case with other disabilities. Parent Teacher Associations and social clubs operating as offshoots of the ATC further reinforced this. Carers, therefore, did not usually have to make themselves visible. Indeed some service providers felt carers were too visible.

Both areas included in the study had begun to implement ideas about normalization, self-advocacy and independent living into ATC provision. The local authority in Area II, for example, no longer referred to ATCs, but to day centres. The emphasis, as described by a manager, was on 'education' and 'improvement' and 'a more community-based provision' such as work placements or courses at local colleges:

> 'We should provide a service which is relevant to the individual and that if a person is capable of a certain type of activity, then really we would be pushing them towards it.'

Most service managers agreed and saw ATCs as outdated and not developing the full potential of the user. Carers, however, valued the integrated and defined care provided by ATCs. They felt secure with this form of provision and found the new forms of day care less appropriate. From the carer's view these changes had three important consequences. First, a more intense but more fragmented provision would reduce their time away from the cared-for person, and disrupt the carer's own day activities. Under the old regime, the cared-for person attended the day centre between 9.00 a.m. and 3.00 p.m. The new forms of provision, however, no longer guarantee such a block of time. Second, carers felt that these changes increased risk as the person with the learning disability moved from placement to placement without supervision. Mrs Trolle said that she would only feel secure if she escorted her sister from one form of community activity to another. Finally, the changes introduce an element of uncertainty about future provision. Someone could move, for example, from an ATC to employment or a different form of day care; whereas service practitioners saw this as appropriate in the development of an individual, carers felt it made for an uncertain future.

Some service providers recognized that the new forms of provision would result in a loss of respite for carers and increased risk, but felt it was a necessary sacrifice to achieve progress. One manager, for example, commented:

> 'So I think at this stage we really have to be a bit ruthless and say look this is the way it's got to go and, yes, there will be some short term reduction, yes we will lose services. We've got to . . . get to a stage where people are getting good services and not creating dependency, where we are not institutionalizing people. We've done that in the past. We are now paying a price for it in terms of lots and lots of people well below their potential.'

It would be wrong, however, to assume that service providers were insensitive to the carers' concerns during these changes. One manager said:

> 'We don't want to upset the families by coming along and after five minutes start making suggestions, you can't do that. They've been going along for years. It would be very insulting. So I try and tell my staff . . . They have to learn to be more diplomatic.'

Indeed many service providers felt that more time should be given to reassuring parents and this should become a priority for services. One manager said:

> 'I think there's an awful lot of work to be done, and reassuring to be done, that we won't be pushing people into situations where they will be unhappy.'

Overnight respite

Both areas offered respite within their hostels and additional placements in the form of holidays were also available. The primary pathway into receiving overnight respite or a holiday placement was through day services. Nearly every person with a learning disability who attended an ATC also received an overnight respite placement. This was usually every two to three months. This pattern, although not a surprising one, caused problems for those carers who would like overnight respite but had no contact with an ATC and their experience illustrates the difficulties that arise when the 'usual' route to overnight respite is not present. Mrs Hurst, for example, whose son did not attend an ATC would have liked some respite. She was, however, unclear how to obtain it and uncertain whether she was eligible: 'I don't know who to discuss it with and nobody tells you.' Other carers faced similar difficulties. While a placement at an ATC does not necessarily solve these problems, it does provide a helpful framework of contact and advice and one that continues over time. It also, of course, usually ensures the visibility of the carer.

As with day care, the overnight respite obtained by a carer was a by-product of a service that aimed to enhance the independence of the cared-for person. The person with the learning disability rather than the carer was, therefore, the focus of provision. One manager felt this fact was too often lost sight of. He believed that when he first joined the area, providing families with 'plenty of breaks' received too much attention. There was, he argued, no consideration of the effect of these breaks on the cared-for person, and they could create longterm problems. The manager, therefore, attempted to reduce the amount of respite offered to carers. Most managers, however, took a more understanding view of the carer's situation and recognized the importance of respite to the carers, particularly when the cared-for person had a profound mental and physical disability. The carers themselves were also more likely to perceive overnight respite as benefiting them rather than a day placement at an ATC.

As we have seen in Chapter 6, many carers regard respite with ambivalence and this applies also to the carers of people with learning disability. Negotiation of the service, therefore, assumed particular importance. Mrs Whitcombe, for example, was grateful to the manager of the ATC for the encouragement he gave. She and her husband had 'soldiered on' for many years before they were finally persuaded to accept respite. A hostel manager showed a similar understanding of the need to negotiate with parents; as a matter of policy, he always arranged a series of visits for prospective residents and their parents. This, he argued, allowed both the carer and the person with the learning disability to get used to the idea of respite gradually.

Carers' acceptance of respite was often conditional and could easily be undermined, even for those for whom it was vital. Mrs Otterburn, for example, only found respite acceptable by convincing herself that her daughter enjoyed the experience. A recent incident when her daughter fell out of bed worried her and brought all her anxieties back: 'If I was being completely honest, I would rather she did not go.' Mrs Whitcombe experienced similar doubts. She cared for her mentally- and physically-disabled daughter. Recently, her daughter had returned from overnight respite with bruises. The carer accepted that her daughter sometimes fell, but was angry that no one at the respite hostel seemed to know how it had happened. This did not stop her using respite but she remarked: 'To be frank, it was no break, worrying myself to death about what was happening to her.'

Social work

Except in arranging a respite placement, few carers had contact with social workers. Although both areas operated specialist social work teams for people with learning disabilities, their caseloads was largely made up of children. Social workers, like other practitioners, felt limited in what they could do for carers of adults with learning disabilities. This was largely because of resource constraints. One social worker, for example, explained that the authority had a limited number of respite beds and she had to ration carers. This issue was central to Mrs Trolle's experience of social work. She was due to go into hospital for an operation and requested a respite placement for her sister. The social worker suggested that Mrs Trolle's husband could care for her sister, but she felt this was inappropriate. She informed social services that they would have to take permanent care of her sister if no place was found. Mrs Trolle and her husband felt they should not have had to make these kinds of threats in order to get respite, and they were critical of the social worker's role in this. Mrs Thomas's experience of social work was more positive. During a respite placement her son had received an eye injury which upset her greatly: 'I just broke down and I was really upset.' Mrs Thomas voiced her concerns to the manager of the ATC who arranged a visit by a social worker. Mrs Thomas appreciated this and 'poured [her] heart out'. She found the social worker understanding and was much reassured.

In general direct social work involvement was rare, with little evidence of social workers acting as mediators between the carer and cared-for, or between other services. Once a placement at an ATC or overnight respite was made, the social worker did not usually maintain contact.

The philosophy of provision

Up to now we have concentrated on the carers' experiences of individual services. But services for people with learning disabilities are organized and managed in the context of particular philosophies of care. These had important consequences for carers, and were often the subject of comment in the interviews.

The principles of normalization, independent living and self-advocacy have achieved wide currency in the field of learning disability. They have been influential in guiding practitioners in their interactions with people with learning difficulties, and in the planning and delivery of services (DHSS 1980; Welsh Office 1983; Audit Commission 1989; DH 1990). These philosophies aim to offer people with learning disabilities choice and independence. They are based on the belief that people with learning difficulties should be socially accepted and valued, with the same rights as other, non-disabled people to live in the mainstream of society as valued and respected citizens (Bank-Mikkelson

1969; Nirje 1970; Sines and Bicknell 1985; Wolfensberger and Thomas 1985; Race 1987).

Normalization is often seen as a positive aspect of service philosophy. The concept, however, encompasses and reflects firmly entrenched social values and beliefs. While challenging certain values and beliefs that are often taken for granted in the form of the negative assumptions about people with learning difficulties, normalization itself makes certain blanket assumptions about what is 'normal' or 'valued' in society. Carers sometimes contest these assumptions. Good practice in the field of learning difficulty aims to encourage people towards assuming an independent adult life. Leaving home, getting a job, having a private sexual life, are seen as significant in achieving this. Carers, however, often regard these aims as unrealistic. Achieving an independent adult life may also marginalize the carer and undermine his or her responsibility and capacity to make decisions about the cared-for person's life. This sense of being responsible is central to how many of the carers perceive their situation.

Current policy and practice increasingly asserts the rights of the individual with the learning disability, usually at the expense of the carers (Hubert 1990; Ward 1990; McGrath 1991; McGrath and Grant 1992). Service managers in Wales, for example, where a comprehensive mental handicap strategy was launched in the 1980s believed that carers had too much say, asserting their own interests rather than those of the person they looked after (McGrath and Grant 1992). This led to ambivalence among professionals about carers' participation in service delivery, and concern lest service provision reflect the needs of the carer rather than the person with the learning disability (McGrath and Grant 1992). Some service providers argue that service delivery for people with learning disabilities should, if not exclude carers, at least reduce their influence. Indeed, this approach is becoming increasingly evident in policy documents which present the role of parents in a negative light, as forming a conservative rather than a progressive force (Ward 1990). Unlike service provision for people with physical disability or mental infirmity, there is the aim, at least in theory, of limiting the influence of the carer and, in extreme forms, of excluding them from service development altogether. This conscious exclusion is a recent development that alters their previous relationship with service provision. Rather than support or underwrite the caregiving relationship, the aim is now to transcend it; the general thrust of policy is towards the model of the superseded carer.

Not surprisingly, carers ofter disagreed with certain principles of normalization, and this could be a major source of conflict between parent-carers and service practitioners, as well as creating tensions between the carer and the cared-for person. Certainly, the carers and service providers interviewed in the study often operated according to different frames of reference. Service practitioners saw a disabled person's well-being in relation to their potential to achieve an independent and 'normal' existence, while emphasizing an individual's right to self-determination. They often described parents as overprotective and not recognizing the full potential of the person they cared for. In general they avoided the term 'carer', preferring to refer to 'parents'. Carers on the other hand, drawing from a different frame of reference, viewed well-being in terms of maintaining the cared-for person's security, reducing risk and of being themselves involved in the decisions about the cared-for person's life. Achieving an independent adult life could, for example, marginalize the carer and undermine his or her responsibility and capacity to make decisions about the cared-for person's life. This was particularly difficult for carers to come to terms with because, as we have seen, a sense of being responsible is central to the experience of many carers. In addition, carers often regarded the aims of normalization and independent living as unrealistic, with many claiming that service practitioners did not have adequate resources to underwrite their ideological aspirations. In general they felt that they were bearing the brunt of the changes, but without the necessary backup from service providers.

The conflict of interest arising from applying the ideas of normalization, independent living and self-advocacy is complex. The relationship involves three people – the carer, the person with the learning disability and service practitioner – each with a different frame of reference. Each one, however, is equally valid. Our account, although giving priority to the carer, does not intend to dismiss the needs of the person with the learning disability.

Conflicting views: a case study

The experience of Mrs Trolle who looked after her sister, Cathy, who had Down's syndrome encapsulates many of the problems that we have been discussing. The case illustrates the different frames of reference employed by carers and service providers as well as pointing to possible tensions that can occur between the carer and the person they look after.

Cathy attended a day centre for people with learning disabilities five days a week. Throughout the interview Mrs Trolle was extremely critical of the day care received by her sister:

> 'They say they want to put them in the community. They want them to go on public transport, they want them to go out and do jobs. Well I don't feel inclined to let her go on public transport because I don't feel she's safe and also I don't want her to go to jobs where there is there any danger with machinery or her having any of these attacks. Sometimes she's overfriendly with strangers and I don't feel, I don't want to let her do these things.'

The carer felt the centre encouraged her sister in ways that gave her unrealistic expectations. These created tension in the relationship:

> 'She thinks they will put her in the flat and she'll have a mortgage and she'll have a wage . . . She blames me because she can't do these things . . . She can't read and write. Now they tell her she can be a secretary . . . They tell her these things because she wants to hear them. All right, they don't want any bother and it's the easiest way out.'

Mrs Trolle felt that these developments had occurred within the last two years. Before this she was much happier with day care provision:

> 'To my mind the old style was so much better . . . Now they've got these younger ones, all they do with them is take them out. They don't teach them anything, they don't have their little jobs. Their attitude is different.'

The manager of the day centre attended by Cathy, however, took a different view. He saw Mrs Trolle as overprotective and not appreciating the potential capabilities of her sister:

> 'She [Cathy] certainly knows her own mind and she does quite a lot of advocating on behalf of some of her peers within the centre and I think she finds that very frustrating when she goes home and it's a case of, "Now sit down, I'll make you a cup of tea. Don't put the kettle on, you might burn yourself", and all this sort of stuff.'

The manager remarked that the carer prevented Cathy from using public transport and objected to her obtaining employment. Indeed Mrs Trolle had threatened to withdraw her sister from the day centre. Working to these restrictions, he felt, meant he was not offering an appropriate service for the cared-for person:

> 'I mean we are here to provide a service for Cathy. We should be respecting Cathy's wishes because she's an adult, but I remember having a conversation with Mrs Trolle and she did threaten to withdraw Cathy from the service if we pursued public transport and so really, like I say, we were between the devil and the deep blue sea on that one.'

In retrospect the manager felt that he could have done more to reassure the carer, but felt the key problem was one of resources:

> 'Obviously we can certainly do better with our communication with Mrs Trolle. Perhaps we ought to put more emphasis upon reassuring Mrs Trolle that Cathy is capable of doing a lot more. But what I don't want to do is promise too much and not have the resources to back it up, you see, which is very difficult.'

Conclusion

The situation of carers of people with learning disabilities, although similar in many ways to that of other carers, is also significantly different. As we have seen, caring here is less a question of physical labour than of 'being responsible' for the cared-for person. The most common relationship is one of parents caring for offspring, and this affects assumptions about the balance of authority between the carer, the cared-for person and the service providers, with parents carrying overexpectations derived from childcare into the adulthood of the cared-for person. There are also significant differences in relation to service provision for this group which has a coherence not found in other service sectors. Services for people with a learning disability are also informed by much stronger service philosophies, and these can lead to significant conflicts between service providers and carers as to how and whether their interests and interpretations should be incorporated into practice.

Chapter 8 *CARERS OF ADULTS WITH MENTAL HEALTH PROBLEMS*

The literature on informal care has not traditionally encompassed the carers of people with mental health problems. Carers who are looking after someone with dementia have always had a prominent place in the literature, but relatives supporting a younger (under 60 years) person with mental health problems have in general been excluded from that 'carer' framework. The relatively little work that has been done on the subject has tended to be undertaken in isolation from the literature on caring and within a different conceptual framework: that of psychiatry (Perring *et al.* 1990).

Mental health terminology is controversial, with different words implying different theoretical stances. We have adopted the term 'mental health problems' to cover the range of difficulties that people experience in the area of mental health. Some of these problems can be conceptualized as mental illness, and we use that term on occasions to distinguish psychotic conditions like schizophrenia.

As we have noted, the traditional conceptualization of caring has been strongly task-focused with activities like lifting, toileting and dressing, seen as the defining feature of care-giving. These physical tasks, however, are rarely of central importance in relation to mental health problems and are commonly absent. As a result, caring for someone with mental health problems is often not regarded as 'caring' at all. In Chapter 1 we suggested that the concept of caring was best seen in terms of a series of elements, no single one of which was defining. Although physical assistance is of relatively little significance in relation to mental health problems, two other elements in the definition are more so: the consequences of sharing your life with someone, and being responsible. Although the sense of 'being responsible' is common to all care-giving, it is particularly central in mental health problems. Providing a home, coping with money or public authorities, managing periodic crises or hospitalization, as well as trying to prevent the cared-for person from falling into lethargy and self-neglect are all part of the responsibilities that carers assume (Perring *et al.* 1990). In the carer's mind the obligation is clear. Many feel that they are responsible for the conduct of their relative, and that they can be blamed or shamed by their actions.

The consequences of sharing your life with someone with mental health problems can be considerable. Mental health problems can disrupt family life and impose a social isolation that reinforces guilt and stigma. Disturbed behaviour can cause distress and social embarrassment. Parents of offspring diagnosed as schizophrenic often find their other children hostile to the sufferer, and this can cause further friction. Carers can become isolated through reluctance to invite people into the home (Johnstone *et al.* 1984; Fadden *et al.* 1987). Spouse carers in particular can find it difficult to maintain a joint social life if one partner is withdrawn and apathetic. In general, carers of people with mental health problems feel they have to cope with a world that does not want to understand their situation, and they can feel lonely and trapped (Kreisman and Joy 1974; Thompson and Doll 1982; Gibbons *et al.* 1984).

As with all disabilities the onset of the problem can be a particularly stressful time in which the carer may have to come to terms with a fundamental change in the person and in the relationship (Creer and Wing 1974; Creer *et al.* 1982). Carers sometimes experience an acute sense of bereavement or loss at this change. Behaviour may have altered to such an extent that they feel they are living with a totally different person. They may be uncertain how to respond, not wanting to be unsympathetic to the person they look after, and yet frustrated, baffled and angry at their behaviour (Fadden *et al.* 1987; Perring *et al.* 1990). Carers may also have to face new responsibilities, taking over areas of life that were previously managed by the other person.

In describing the consequences of looking after someone with mental health problems, it is important to note that there is no single mental illness, and different types of mental health problems have different consequences and meanings for carers. There is an important distinction to be drawn between schizophrenic and other psychotic conditions on the one hand and neurotic conditions on the other. Psychotic conditions are seen more as 'mind disorders' involving impairment of cognitive functioning, particularly in relation to perception and thinking; and they normally imply an absence of insight. These conditions can involve difficult behaviour, such as aggression, mood swings, lack of motivation and withdrawal (Grad and Sainsbury 1963; Creer and Wing 1974; Creer 1975; Vaughn and Leff 1976, 1981; Fadden *et al.* 1987) Mrs Brearley's son, for example, spent day after day lying on his bed, refusing to wash and listening to loud rock music. On occasions he was violent and had smashed the windows of a local church. Neurotic conditions on the other hand are characterized by feelings of depression or anxiety and by obsessive, compulsive or phobic behaviour. People who are diagnosed as neurotic can show a range of behaviour including threatened or attempted suicide, crying, extreme anxiety, withdrawn behaviour with no inclination to speak, obsessive or hypochondriacal preoccupations. Mrs Walker's husband, for example, became severely depressed and anxious in the wake of redundancy, and made a suicide attempt. Mr Gibson has experienced similar bouts of severe depression and had battered his wife.

Mental health problems can be episodic in character. This is particularly true of conditions like schizophrenia where the sufferer may experience bouts of florid behaviour interspersed with periods of stability (Creer and Wing 1974), though it can apply also to depression. The variable nature of the condition means that the carer's needs will also fluctuate. Carers may not require support from services for several months, but then need immediate help at the onset of crisis.

Is mental illness different?

Seeing the supporter of someone with mental health problems within the 'carer' framework brings advantages. It frees the subject from an excessively psychiatric perspective which tends to see carers as part of the social background of the patient and rarely focuses on their circumstances *per se*. It allows helpful parallels to be drawn. But are there issues of a more ontological nature that mean that caring in relation to mental health problems is different? The most obvious of these turns around the question of causality. Are 'carers' implicated in the mental health problems that their relatives experience in ways that make the application of that framework inappropriate? Are they causers as well as carers? In relation to schizophrenia the argument arises most clearly out of the work of Laing and others fashionable in the 1960s that saw the origins of schizophrenia as lying in the family, particularly in the behaviour of 'schizophrenogenic mothers' (Bateson *et al.* 1956; Laing 1960; Lidz 1968). These theories have largely been laid aside as an explanation of the condition, though they live on in some professional and lay conceptions of the illness and can affect the way carers are perceived. Perhaps of greater current significance in structuring the responses of service providers to relatives, however, has been the theory of expressed emotion (Kuipers 1979; Falloon *et al.* 1982). This approach, though it does not necessarily regard the family as the source of the illness, does see the behaviour of relatives as potentially implicated in the precipitation of crises. Research has associated families where there are high levels of expressed emotion with relapse and a poorer prognosis for the patient (Brown *et al.* 1972; Vaughn and Leff 1976; Falloon *et al.* 1982).

Despite the presence of these interpretations that implicate families in, at least, the course of the illness, schizophrenia is in many ways the easiest form of mental illness to which to apply a carer framework. Schizophrenia is often regarded as the paradigmatic mental illness, the condition that approaches nearest the medical model of mental health problems as a form of 'illness'. This endows it with an objective, neutral quality that parallels that of physical illness or disability. It is an illness that has consequences, rather than one that has meaning (Sontag 1983). It can be seen as something that has simply occurred, and the relationship is not implicated in it. As a result it is easier to place schizophrenia within the same 'carer' framework as physical disability or learning difficulties.

With other mental health problems such as depression the issues are less clear-cut. There has been a wide recognition, from the work of Brown and his colleagues onwards, of the role of psychosocial factors in depression (Brown and Harris 1978). Indeed many would argue that such problems are best interpreted as arising out of social circumstances with which the individual is unable to cope rather than mental 'illness' as such. Among these circumstances can be the family and marital relationships of the 'cared-for' person; this puts a question mark over the appropriateness of the term 'carer'. Family systems theories, whereby the sufferer is seen as the bearer of symptoms that belong to the family as a whole, further disrupt the automatic application of the 'carer' paradigm to these situations. It is not appropriate in a work of this scope to enter into the debates concerning the causes of mental illness, except to note that they have implications for the ways in which carers are seen by service providers. It was certainly the case that we as researchers faced greater ambiguity in relation to classifying carers in this group, compared with the other client or patient categories, both in the sense of ambiguity as to who was the carer and who the cared-for, and uncertainty as to whether the relationship should be classified as one of caring.

Carers of whom?: diagnosis and relationship

In the study sample, diagnosis overlapped heavily with relationship. The majority of people diagnosed as schizophrenic were cared for by a parent. By contrast, the majority of spouses cared for someone with severe depression or with a mixed or unclear diagnosis. The overlap between relationship and diagnosis had important consequences for how the situation was conceived by both the carer and service providers. In the case of spouses with depression, the situation was often interpreted in terms of marital problems; issues of the meaning of the illness, the potential conflict of interest and the possible ending of care were seen within that framework. Although by the nature of the study, these spouses had all remained in the relationship, two couples separated shortly after the interview and a third was considering doing so. This was in marked contrast to the spouse carers of other client groups, where there was no serious thought of separation (except in the case of a small number of elderly spouses who were not considering separation as such but the institutional care of their spouse). The pattern raises the question of whether mental health problems breach the obligations of marriage in ways that other illnesses do not. There are certain parallels with the effect of brain injury or dementia, both of which entail a loss of the person in ways that can weaken the ties of marriage. But mental health problems entail an additional aspect. Illnesses like depression pose questions of intersubjective meaning that are different in character from those of physical disability, where the disability has a neutral quality to it and has, as it were, descended on the relationship by mischance. With depression the separation between the condition and the relationship is harder for the carer to maintain; it is difficult to objectify the symptoms of the illness which can all too easily be interpreted as meaningful, and thus experienced as anger, malignity or coldness.

In the case of parents of children diagnosed as schizophrenic, the overlap between relationship and condition produced a set of issues that had much in common with those posed by learning disability. Schizophrenia, although not a congenital condition, often manifests itself in the teens or twenties, before the sufferer has established an independent life as an adult. As a result between 60 and 70 per cent of people diagnosed as schizophrenic will return from a first admission to hospital to live with their family (Goldman 1980). This pattern of onset affects what we term the 'moral status' of the sufferer (see Chapter 9), although to a lesser degree than is the case where the condition has been present from birth. Conflicts over adulthood, the transitions to independent living and the problems of securing a decent future for the person after the lifetime of the parent are central issues for this group.

Mental health services

The majority of services for this group are found within the health sector. This was particularly true in the past, when almost no services for people with mental health difficulties existed in the community or outside a medical remit. Despite some developments towards a more social-care focus involving the social services and voluntary sectors, the predominance of health services has remained. The trend of thinking on community care in the last decade has retained the idea that people with mental health problems are in some sense different from other community care clients and that mental illness 'belongs' more appropriately with the health sector. Indeed, the influential Audit Commission report of 1986 assigned this client group to health services, and later policy developments such as the mental illness specific grant have endorsed the idea that mental illness should be seen as apart, and within a predominantly medical framework. The dominance of the health service and the medical model has, of course, been vigorously challenged by those who would both like to see an alternative perspective on the mental health problems that people experience, and who wish to emphasize the social as opposed to medical needs of sufferers. We shall return to these issues when we discuss services that operate on a social work model.

Services for people with mental health difficulties lack the integrated character that we noted in relation to learning difficulties. This is partly because people in this category form a less clearly-defined group. As we have seen, planning in relation to learning difficulties has the advantage that the group being planned for is relatively small, comparatively well defined and usually known to service providers. This is not so with mental illness, where people recover and move in and out of the orbit of services, and where many wish to avoid contact with psychiatric services altogether.

We will first discuss services that have a medical focus: these include consultant psychiatrists and community psychiatric nurses. We shall then turn to services organized by the local authority, examining in particular the role of the social worker. Finally, we shall explore the issue of respite.

Services with a medical focus

As we have seen in earlier sections on general practitioners and hospital consultants, medicine focuses on the individual patient and on the medical aspects of his or her needs. This is true also of psychiatric medicine. The predominant approach within the psychiatric services is that of seeing carers as 'relatives', as part of the social background of the patient. At times psychiatrists adopted a slightly more 'carer' orientation but, as we shall see, their approach remained predominantly instrumental.

Consultants and carers

Psychiatrists tended to marginalize carers less than did their colleagues in physical medicine. They were more likely to have met the carer but it was clear that the importance they assigned to this related not to the potential needs of the carer but to a wish to gain information about the patient, whether in the form of factual clarification about the past or knowledge of the social and emotional context in which he or she was living. Many carers were happy to provide this information, though one carer of a severely depressed spouse commented rather bitterly on this approach, describing how she was called in by the psychiatrist: 'He asked only a few questions and then said, "I don't want to ask you any more. Just seeing you is all I want."'

Not all psychiatrists saw initial contact with the family solely in terms of gaining information. One emphasized the importance of the initial contact with relatives at the time of the first episode of mental illness, particularly schizophrenia. It was the start of what could be a long-term relationship with the patient and the family. Handling that episode with sensitivity was of great importance: 'Because ultimately you need the relatives on your side to provide the care.' Such an approach was valued by carers. Mrs Mason, the mother of a son diagnosed as schizophrenic, praised the consultant: 'I mean you walk in there and he'll sit and he'll talk as long as you like.'

Consultants, however, sometimes recognized that they were not always the best person to speak to the carer – a view endorsed by some of the carers themselves. Mr Fortner described how the consultants did not talk to him in language he could understand. He would ask a question and they would reply: 'In three or four great big long words and that was complete, and I wouldn't understand.'

Some consultants felt that talking to the carer was something that community psychiatric nurses were particularly effective at doing. Employing them in this role, however, diverted resources that were already hard pressed, and there was little evidence that consultants used them extensively in this way.

In general, psychiatrists showed sympathy for the situation of carers, although the subject was not one about which they had thought extensively. In the interviews they showed an imaginative understanding of what it was like to live with someone with mental health problems, but at the same time they were clear where their principal obligation lay – with the patient – and their sympathetic understanding did not appear to have significant implications for their practice. The emphasis on the patient at times resulted in the exclusion of the carer from information and contact. Consultants felt they had to respect the confidences of the patient, particularly where the carer's role in the situation was unclear. One psychiatrist made a distinction in his practice between the carers of 'psychotics' and 'neurotics'. With neurotics he felt he had to respect the confidentiality of the doctor–patient relationship, and could only talk to or involve the spouse or other carer if the patient wanted him to do so:

'Now with psychotic illness, we are in a slightly different situation, because of the illness. We are aware that their welfare is depending on other people, and other people may have to be drawn in.'

Though the doctor–patient relationship was still important, the demands of confidentiality were less absolute. The consultant felt he had to be able to draw in the family, and in doing this he clearly made a distinction between the 'moral status' of the two types of patient.

The strong focus on the patient was illustrated in the way consultants responded to questions concerning the conflict of interest and the possibility of the ending of care. As one psychiatrist commented:

'My job is to explain to them and they have to make the decision . . . it is up to them to choose. Certainly I would try very hard to make them understand what's happening to that person.'

When probed as to what he would do if the situation was harming the carer, but not the patient, he replied: 'I can see the background, but I will do nothing about it . . .' He went on to emphasize that his duty was to the patient. The exchange illustrates well a characteristic combination of sympathetic understanding for the carer but a clear focus on the patient.

Sometimes consultants were in conflict with the wishes of the family. This arose most often in relation to parents of offspring diagnosed as schizophrenic. There are clear parallels with the situation in learning difficulties, although the conflicts were not so overt, nor fuelled by so strong an ideology. Consultants, in wishing their schizophrenic patients to live more independently, were governed by three principal ideas. The first was a model of *normal growing up* whereby children achieve adulthood through a process of separation and individuation. The second incorporated a notion of *handicap*. Though schizophrenia was seen by the consultants as producing the patient's primary problems, they recognized that they suffered in addition from difficulties not caused by the illness itself, but by people's attitudes to it and the social circumstances that surrounded sufferers. Among these circumstances could be overprotective parents who prevented the patients from achieving the independence of which they were capable. Last, there was the idea of the *future*. Here offspring with schizophrenia were in the same situation as were those with learning disabilities and psychiatrists usually wanted to see their patients making the transition to independent living before it was forced by circumstances. Where the carer of the patient with schizophrenia was a spouse, however, the attitude of the consultants was different – they assumed the continuing interdependence of the couple and appeared happier to regard the relationship as one of 'caring'.

The wish to see offspring living an independent life had consequences for the attitude that consultants took to certain carers. Mrs Hobson, for example, was an elderly widow caring for her son diagnosed as schizophrenic. Though the consultant described it as a very caring relationship, he believed that David would be better off away from his mother, standing on his own feet – something he felt with support he could do. She was herself quite frail, with very bad eyesight and a heart condition, and she relied on her son for company and emotional support. The consultant was not aware of the full extent of her physical problems, and was reluctant to encourage her emotional needs. When asked whether he saw her as a carer or not his reply was equivocal, and reflected his reluctance to endorse her in this role. From her viewpoint, however, this stance meant that she experienced the consultant as someone who was indifferent to her problems and 'did not seem to bother to talk to me'.

A second example involved a mother caring for both a daughter diagnosed as schizophrenic and son with some form of psychosis. Once again, the psychiatrist saw the relationships as overdependent, and he wanted to encourage the children to be more independent of their mother. She had, however, 'sabotaged' several attempts to achieve this: removing the son from the rehabilitation ward and walking out of family therapy. In the psychiatrist's perception she needed her caring to make sense of her life. At various times she had made 'cries for help' in the form of a suicide attempt and drinking and she felt ignored and unsupported by the psychiatric service. This was in a sense true, since as the psychiatrist explained: 'I've always taken the view that we shouldn't be supporting Mum to look after John.'

By and large, psychiatrists did not intervene between the carer and cared-for person overtly. They acted in a negative way, by not reinforcing the relationship and sometimes by ignoring the views of carers.

Community psychiatric nurses and carers

Although the community psychiatric nurses (CPNs) were identified by some consultants as an appropriate group to talk to and work with carers, such involvement was rare. The work of the community nursing service in both areas followed a pattern familiar from the literature whereby the bulk of its activity turned around providing injections and ensuring compliance with medication. A number of carers commented rather negatively on the way that CPNs were in and out of the house without stopping to talk to them or the cared-for person.

The injection focus did not appear to operate, as it did for carers of older mentally infirm people, as a focal intervention that triggered other aspects of the nurses' support. In so far as CPNs did stop to talk – and this appeared relatively rare – the focus was clearly on the patient and not the carer. In part, this arose from the fact that it was possible to have a conversation with the patient, something that was rarely the case with dementia and where the carer as a result benefited from the direct attention of the nurse. Carers of younger people with mental health problems thus appeared to get *less* support from the CPNs than did those of older people. The difference was reiterated in relation to carer support groups by a CPN who contrasted his practice with that of the elderly team who organized carer support groups, something he felt was 'unnecessary' for his client group. The focus on the patient also arose from the fact that in both areas the service was described as being under pressure, and although some CPNs would have liked to have been able to offer a service to carers, doing so came low in their priorities and was displaced by work with patients. For one CPN carers were effectively invisible. He initially stated in the interview that few of his patients lived with anyone, but was forced to modify this when he went through his caseload and found that 25 out of 44 in fact did so. (Wolsey, quoted in Brooker 1990 found that in one regional health authority people diagnosed as schizophrenic and living with family constituted a third of the case load of generic CPNs.) When asked if this knowledge would change his response, he replied:

> 'No. I respond as needs be. I won't look and see if I can find someone to work with. I will respond, not necessarily to crises, but if people say there is a problem, I will attend to it. One thing I don't do is going looking for problems to attend to, unlike some.'

Though no carer received extensive support from a CPN, two did have some contact. These were both cases involving spouses who were depressed. Because the spouses had problems that could be seen within a marital therapy framework, the carers were included within the ambit of the CPNs' work in a way that did not seem to occur when they were simply seen as carers. One CPN did articulate a more active involvement, describing carers as 'co-therapists'. In this, however, he was like the consultants, seeing carers as a source of information as well as individuals who could be encouraged to behave in more therapeutic ways. He expressed a wish to help carers themselves, but he recognized that his ultimate responsibility lay with the patient: that was the 'bottom line'.

There has been a growing interest in recent years in the idea of 'psycho-education', in the sense of the systematic provision of information and advice to relatives (Barrowclough and Tarrier 1984). Although the approach does produce a focus on carers it does so in a highly instrumental way with interventions seen as a means of improving the situation of the patient and with little recognition of the impact of the condition on the relatives' lives or of the need to alleviate their burdens. We did not have any examples of such activity in our sample. Indeed, some of the carers like Mrs Brealey commented on how they had learned by trial and error the best way to handle their son's behaviour, and they would have welcomed more concrete advice. Optimistic accounts of the work of CPNs that have stressed their potential educational role in relation to carers were not borne out by the cases in the study.

Services within a social work tradition

As we have noted, services for people with mental health problems are predominantly provided within the health sector, and within a strong medical paradigm. Despite this, social services still regard themselves as having a distinctive role to play in relation to this client group. This partly involves a different approach to therapy and support – one rooted in the psychodynamic traditions of counselling – and partly emphasizing the social care needs of clients for help with practical matters like housing, benefits and employment. In practice, social services departments offer a limited service to these clients. One social work manager, for example, believed they offered a social work service to people with mental health problems rather than a comprehensive service based on a social care perspective. This was something he regretted and he recognized that the health authority was in practice the lead authority for this client group.

The dominance of health care professionals was perceived by social work managers as resulting in a narrow focus on the patient, which they contrasted with the broader social work tradition. The manager commented how in his work he had always taken a family focus, whereas health authority staff:

> 'Deal with the patient. The family is an appendage. Make a nuisance of themselves . . . we are much more conscious of people being part of a family dynamic, and you can't separate them out. It seems easier for nurses to see people as quite distinct from their families . . . that has been a tension.'

This contrast was in general borne out in the cases in the study.

Social work and carers

Social workers in both areas were aware that the carers of people with mental health problems were a low priority group. As a manager in Area I explained, carers came after clients, and clients came: 'Third, fourth or fifth, or twenty-third in terms of priority for local authority resources.' Pressure of work meant that support for carers got pushed to the back of the queue. As a specialist social worker at the community mental health centre commented:

> 'When your time is up to here, and you know you don't do as well as you ought, you have a kind of ideal in your mind and you don't achieve it, either with clients or their relatives, sometimes I suspect the relatives do get the short straw. They are regarded as having more resources somehow than the ill person.'

Social workers, like other practitioners, felt they were limited in what they could do in relation to carers. Mrs Brealey was caring for her son diagnosed as schizophrenic, but his behaviour had got to the point when she wanted him to leave, and she approached the consultant who referred Adam to the local social work team. The social worker arranged for him to go to a hostel run by a charity. The placement soon broke down because of Adam's behaviour associated with his drinking. The social worker felt that the hostel staff had overreacted and failed to respond professionally:

> 'Here's Mr and Mrs Brealey, an elderly couple who coped with it, God knows how many years, and here's the agency which is supposed to be offering a professional service and the minute there's a hiccup, 'Get him out of here.' I mean it's ridiculous . . . It annoys me when I hear professionals discharging their responsibilities on to the parents, we're there to offer a service, either we offer it or we get the hell out of it.'

There was no suggestion at this point that his mother should resume responsibility for his care, and another placement was found.

In general social workers focused less exclusively on the client than did the consultants, and they appeared to be more aware of the conflicts of interest involved in caring than were the CPNs. As we shall see, some of them were involved in complex negotiations between the parties and these were not confined to marital cases. Social workers also appeared to be more willing to contemplate the ending of care-giving and their own role in enabling this, were this to be the wish of the carer. In relation to offspring diagnosed as schizophrenic, social workers had the same aspirations for their independence as did the consultants, though the issue played a less marked role in their practice. This was mainly because the majority of such cases were managed by hospital-based services and there was no strong referral pathway leading to social work involvement.

Social workers could find themselves acting as mediators between the carer and the cared-for, as well as between the carer and other services. A social worker had become involved with Mrs Harrison over an incident at a hostel where her son who was diagnosed as schizophrenic was living. The hostel had been established as a 'haven', with a philosophy of 'peace' and a strong emphasis on self-determination. The social worker was not unsympathetic to this, but she believed that the hostel operated a policy of 'excluding relatives', and this tendency was reinforced in Patrick's case by his telling his key worker that his problems came from his mothers' interference. As a result, they excluded her from information, and refused to tell her about a suicide attempt that Patrick made. Patrick came off his drugs, possibly with the encouragement of the key worker, and at some point stopped eating adequately. When the social worker called at the hostel she saw that he was in a seriously psychotic state, overruled the hostel staff and had him compulsorily admitted to hospital. At this point both Patrick and Mrs Harrison became her clients. Mrs Harrison was very angry at what had happened and was creating a lot of 'trouble' on the ward, where staff saw her as interfering and overbearing:

> 'The other mental, clinical team were saying, "Patrick's our patient, we listen to Patrick," and Patrick, who was then much better, "Patrick decides his own future."'

The social worker understood Mrs Harrison's anxieties but saw how counterproductive they were:

> 'I saw my role on the ward round, if possible, trying to represent her view, but not in such a way as to antagonize even further the people on the ward who deal with Patrick.'

The situation was complex, and this account does not do justice to all the factors involved. It provides an example, however, of how social workers are called to balance the interests of carer and cared-for and act not just as counsellors but also mediators with other services. The case was an unfortunate one where things went badly wrong, and we do not want to suggest that this was the inevitable consequence of progressive approaches. It does illustrate however, the tensions that can arise when staff pursue a strong policy of self-determination. Whether Mrs Harrison had a 'right' to know about her son's suicide attempt is open to debate. It was clear, however, that the policy caused considerable distress to her, and in her view violated rights implicit in her relationship. The social worker was very much aware of the dilemmas posed by the wish to underwrite the independence of clients:

> 'How does one square the demands the carer's making for information with the patient's expressed wish not to give them that information? . . . [the

local voluntary group] have a lot of dissatisfied relatives who have been at the receiving end of lack of information because of that particular policy.'

The problem of respite

Respite is almost wholly absent as a concept within the mental health sector. This is in clear contrast to the other client groups where respite is a familiar concept and one recognized as of central importance in the support of carers. Not surprisingly, many carers would have welcomed some form of respite. Mrs Hobson described how difficult it was living with her son, David, who was either under her feet in their small flat or, if out on his own, a source of anxiety, and she wished he could be persuaded to go to a day centre. Other carers would have liked to have been able to go away on holiday, but felt they could not leave their son or spouse uncared for and alone in the house. They were fearful of a crisis, of some dangerous act, or simply of decline and self-neglect. Mrs Bourne, for example, in her interview had said that she would be happy to go away if a flexible visiting service could be arranged for her husband that would ensure that he took his medication and kept an eye on him. The clearest expressions of desire for respite arose in relation to schizophrenia. One mother, active in a mental illness association, asserted that there was no essential difference in this regard between learning disability and mental illness: respite for carers was just as appropriate.

Why then was it largely unavailable and, indeed, unfamiliar as concept in this field? The issue turns around the relative autonomy of the cared-for person in making choices and enforcing them. The majority of people with mental health problems have no wish to go into overnight respite, particularly when it is available only on hospital wards. As one consultant explained, most simply do not perceive of themselves as a burden on their families, and remain unaware of the strain caused by their illness. They regard themselves as capable and see no reason why they should go onto a ward if their parents or family want to go away. With other client groups, the carer is able to exert greater control. In relation to someone with senile dementia, for example, the combination of their lack of mental competence and their physical dependence allows both carers and service providers to override to some degree the unwillingness of the cared-for person to attend day care or go into respite. This is not the case with mental health problems where the sufferer is usually under no physical constraint, and is able to be out in the community as he or she wishes.

Service providers in the mental health field respond to this, endorsing the autonomy of their patients and encourage them towards greater independence. Respite operates in contradiction to these wishes. Good psychiatric care involves responding to the patient as an individual and endorsing their capacity to make choices. Trying to force them to attend a day hospital or go into respite against their wishes is in direct conflict with this, and something few practitioners would want to do. Sometimes the reluctance of service providers to provide respite arose from their inability to identify it as a problem for the carer. Mr Marwood, for example, caring for his brother wanted some form of respite. The CPN appeared to have a good grasp of the situation and his account agreed with that of Mr Marwood, except that he was unaware of this wish; he went on in the interview to state that he could think of no carers who wanted respite except those caring for someone with dementia. In a similar way a social worker at the community mental health centre stated rather flatly that he did not go into cases where respite was a problem.

Day-time respite

Day care was provided in the two authorities in a range of settings: day hospitals, a specialist day centre run by social services, a voluntary centre, a community mental health centre and drop-in facilities. In neither area, however, did practitioners regard this as adequate and they were aware how the pattern of provision either failed to meet the needs of certain patient/clients or resulted in the inappropriate use of facilities. Davis (1984) suggests that this uneven, *ad hoc*, pattern of provision is characteristic of day care in this sector.

None of the staff at these facilities saw the provision of respite for carers as the purpose of a placement. Some managers recognized that attendance could bring that benefit, but their perception of this was much weaker than was the case with the other client groups. The manager of the specialist day centre run by social services recognized that about half of the attenders lived with relatives and for about seven of these (out of 37 attenders) the centre did have a respite function, but she emphasized that selection and attendance were determined only by the capacity of the cared-for person to benefit from the programmes. None of the day centres in the mental health sector had chosen to start a carer support group, though this was a common feature in day centres for other client groups.

Much day care in the mental health field was 'voluntary' by nature, where users attended at will. Here the crucial issue turned around providing a form of activity that was sufficiently stimulating and enjoyable to attract users by choice, for as we have commented above, this was a group who could exercise choice and that fact had implications for carers. Mrs Hobson, for example, would have liked her son to attend a centre to give her a break from his presence in the flat or her anxieties about his behaviour. He had attended the day hospital and the local voluntary centre but was bored:

> 'He had nothing to do. He was sitting there. That's what made him not go back . . . I do miss it. He could do with something to do.'

The problem of providing good-quality day occupation was reflected in the comments of both consultants and social services managers. As one manager remarked in relation to the day hospital: 'You can take horses to the water but at least half of them won't drink.' He felt the needs of people with mental health problems were more individual:

> 'You can't plan in that systematic way that you can in mental handicap by and large, where you can assume that although there will be the odd people who will feel the service is inappropriate, the majority will continue.'

In the eyes of most service providers, the ideal form of day occupation was employment, though one manager believed that this was easier to obtain for people with learning difficulties than those with mental illness. Employers, he explained, were interested in reliability more than ability, and people with mental illness tended to have the second rather than the first. One carer, Mr Palmer, had obtained an interesting day occupation for his son Mike outside the mental illness sector though using Manpower Services Commission (MSC) funded employment training. Though schizophrenia was a new field to the manager of the scheme, she did some reading on the subject and appeared to take having Mike in her stride. She was relaxed about his parents' involvement, and said that she had not found them difficult, as some service providers had suggested she might.

Overnight respite

Overnight respite posed more problems than did day respite. A social services manager accepted that this was a 'big gap', since they could offer 'virtually nothing' except hospital admission. Consultant psychiatrists did sometimes use beds in this way, but only in relation to people with a psychotic illness. One consultant said he had used both acute and rehabilitation beds to give relatives a break. Another consultant was more circumspect in his comments. When asked about the case of Mr Bourne who was diagnosed as schizophrenic and whose wife had expressed a wish for respite in the interview, he explained that there was no place that he could appropriately go. He would not admit him to the ward, partly because of pressure on beds but also because he had no need of hospital care, and there was no other appropriate accommodation available locally. Mr Bourne, would anyway refuse to go, he pointed out, since one of his delusions was that his wife had another man and wanted to get rid of him.

A number of service providers on both the social services and health sides expressed the wish for some more flexible form of respite provision based around the kind of fostering or sitting services that have been developed for other client groups. Olsen and Rolf (1984) have reviewed the provision and effectiveness of boarding out or substitute family care for mentally ill people, but they do not discuss its use for respite. One hostel worker believed that there might be difficulties in recruiting volunteers willing to work with mentally ill people.

Conclusion

Caring for someone with mental health problems has not normally been included in accounts of care-giving; mental illness tends to be seen as 'different'. There are indeed differences. It is harder, for example, to objectify the condition and separate it from the relationship. Carers may also at times be implicated in the condition, or at least its manifestation. There are, however, good reasons for incorporating them within a carer framework. The balance of activity may be different, with greater emphasis on 'being responsible' and the consequences of sharing your life with a disabled person and less on physical tasks, but there are enough similarities in the situation for it to be appropriately seen as 'caring'. It is also the case that service providers respond to factors that are common to caring, such as moral status, relationship and the existence of a future, and that these mediate how they conceptualize the situation and what they regard as an appropriate service response. Carers, however, tend to be neglected in service delivery. The services they are in contact with are predominantly medical and emphasize the individual patient and the medical aspect of their needs. Services are also concerned to encourage the independence of the patient rather than endorse their dependence on their relatives.

Chapter 9 *MEDIATING*

This chapter explores the factors mediating between carers and service receipt, analysing the systematic assumptions relating to the carer or the caring relationship that structure service response. We start with factors at the individual level, exploring the significance of the attitude that a carer adopts to his or her caring role, and the impact of the views of the cared-for person and other kin. We then move to more normatively-laden factors such as relationship, the existence or otherwise of a future beyond the caring relationship, and what we term the 'moral status' of the cared-for person. Finally, we discuss those factors operating at a social structural level, such as gender, age, class and race. Although we draw these out as separate elements, they are interactive. Gender, for example, affects the responses that carers adopt to their role. Relationship interacts with 'moral status' to determine how far carers can or ought to control the situation. We explore these interactions further below.

Before turning to the mediating factors, it is helpful to recap briefly on two features of caring that affect the ways in which carers operate. Caring is embedded in kinship and marital relationships. This central fact affects how society, public agencies, service providers and the carers themselves interpret the meaning of what is happening and the appropriate relationship of services to it. What sorts of difficulties are deserving of help? What is the picture of normal life that caring can be seen to have disrupted in such a way as to deserve redress? When can carers reasonably feel that they have done enough, and that they deserve relief? The mediating categories that we discuss below affect these kinds of judgments. What we present therefore are factors that structure assumptions about the forms of help that are regarded as legitimate – or perhaps better in this context as 'appropriate', since this is a form of discourse in which the moral assumptions underlying the response are only weakly articulated. Many of the factors we describe – such as age or relationship – are not overtly seen as moral categories, but simply as part of the common-sense social reality that service providers need to relate to in their work.

It will, we hope, be clear that we are not providing an account in terms of the needs-related characteristics of individual carers. Needs-related characteristics focus on factors such as the presence of incontinence, or behavioural difficulties, or measures of stress suggestive of psychiatric intervention or care collapse. The discourse of needs-related characteristics is formed by the conjunction of the tradition of practice with research data; and classic examples of the approach are to be found in the work of Davies and his colleagues (Davies and Challis 1986; Davies *et al.* 1990). We are not suggesting that service providers ignore such practice triggers, or that they are irrelevant to judgments about service provision. We are, however, suggesting that they exist within a context of interpretation that relates to how caring is constructed socially and that in turn structures expectations concerning appropriate service intervention. Needs-related characteristics are mediated through assumptions concerning the meaning of relationships and situations. These are the subject of this chapter.

The second point to recapitulate is that service provision is the product of negotiation. As we explored in Chapter 2, service delivery is to some degree a two-way affair. Whether or not a user or carer receives help can be the result of their own expectations, values and assumptions. It can be affected by how they see their caring and to what extent they regard it as legitimate or appropriate to receive help. If home care is, as has sometimes been suggested, provided on a gender-biased basis, this can be a result of the expectations of users and carers and not simply of service providers and agencies. As we have seen, carers sometimes refuse forms of help that they regard as intrusive, disruptive of their relationship, or otherwise inappropriate. By contrast, some carers – a minority – regard support as something they have a right to, and will make demands on agencies on that basis. What carers expect and what they think it legitimate or appropriate to have help with affects how they respond to service providers, and the degree to which they will themselves seek help. Service provision is thus a result of negotiation between the parties.

Of course, we need to recognize that carers construct their expectations of services in the context of what they are told and what is provided. As we noted earlier, it would be wrong to see the relationship of carers and service providers as an equal one. It is a relationship of power in which the service providers have control over the definitions and the interpretation of the situation as well as over the final allocation. It is still useful, however, to recognize that allocation is in some degree a two-way process of negotiation. The mediating factors that we explore below, therefore, need to be seen from both sides: they structure the expectations of both carers and service providers.

In looking at the operation of these mediating factors on both sides we recognize that their interpretation will vary as between service providers and lay people. Lay and professional logics are different; there is a body of literature that has explored the disjunction between the two (Robinson 1978; Rojeck *et al.* 1988; Oliver 1990). What is notable in this context, however, is the degree to which assumptions were shared. Service providers and carers to a large degree share a common culture about the nature of families and marriage. Of course, as we shall see, there were also differences, for example concerning gender and the degree to which it should underwrite different responsibilities, though differences over this were as prominent between service providers themselves as between service providers and carers. There were, however, some differences that related more directly to service cultures. As we have seen, this was particularly so in the field of learning disabilities. We now turn to the first of the mediating factors, exploring how this structures the negotiation and provision of services.

Factors at the individual level

The attitude of carers to their caring role

We found that carers' responses to their role fell into three main modes: that of engulfment, of balancing/boundary setting and of symbiosis.

The engulfment mode

Engulfment is the mode of response where the carer subordinates his or her life to that of the cared-for person. Caring becomes the centre of their life, and the defining feature of self-identity. It was hard for such carers to distance themselves from the situation and their emotional identification with the cared-for person was often so close that they found it difficult to separate themselves from the cared-for person's pain and suffering.

For which categories of carers was this the dominant response? There tended, not surprisingly, to be an association between mode of response and objectively observable burden. It is difficult not to become engulfed when faced with double incontinence, bizarre behaviour or nightly disturbance. But the association was not total. There were carers whose dominant response was one of engulfment but whose observable 'burden' was low. In these cases, other factors such as the long-term dynamics of the marriage, or a continuing guilt engendered in relation to the birth of a child with disabilities, underwrote the response. Physical pain experienced by the cared-for person also contributed to the likelihood of the carer being engulfed by the situation, since this was an experience from which it was hard for carers to detach themselves.

The response appeared to be a gendered one. More female than male carers fell into this category; the pattern was clearest where the woman was also a spouse. We will explore the impact of gender more fully below, and only refer briefly to an aspect of its operation that has particular relevance to the engulfed mode. Gilligan (1982) in her influential study suggests that males and females have different developmental paths. With males this centres around the achievement of separation from the mother. Females by contrast in achieving maturity are not required to separate themselves from their mothers: the parent who is most closely involved in their development is the same-sex parent with whom they identify. As a result Gilligan argues, males exhibit problems over relatedness and view intimacy as a threat, while females have problems over individuation and experience separation as a threat. Gilligan argues that these differences underwrite the different moral voices of the two genders: that of men cast in terms of the assertion of rights, subject to 'rational' public scrutiny; that of women is cast in terms of responsibilities that are private, negotiated and sensitive to the interests of all involved. Such psychodynamic factors are not of course the only ones structuring the responses of the sexes to caring and in the section on gender we will explore other important elements. However, Gilligan's work does highlight important issues in relation to individuation and autonomy that have particular relevance to the question of engulfment. Many of the features characteristic of this mode of response have their roots in issues of separation. Carers in this category often have difficulty in establishing autonomy for themselves and for their interests; this pattern carries over into their response to receiving service help. The link with gender was not an absolute one. There were instances of male carers who could be described as engulfed, and there were, as we shall see in the next section, some female carers who adopted a more detached and balancing mode. The overlap was, however, striking.

What were the consequences of this mode of response for the negotiation and acceptance of services? The first relates to visibility. Many carers in this category remained invisible to service providers, obscured behind the needs of the person they looked after. They often found it difficult to articulate, or even envisage, their own needs as carers. Accepting help that was primarily aimed at them rather than the cared-for person was difficult, and sometimes seen as a threat to the relationship. Second, many of these carers had so made their lives around caring that they had no alternative occupation or focus. Many did not, or could not, work; as a result they had no activity that could legitimate their asking for relief or allow them to enjoy it. Outings or holidays on their own brought little pleasure; this was particularly a problem for spouses, many of whom had few expectations of social life beyond marriage and who thus shared the limitations imposed by the illness or disability on their spouse. Third, for some the sense of responsibility was so total that they could not share it. Asking for help was seen as an admission of failure. This was particularly associated with mothers of congenitally-disabled offspring or those with learning disabilities. Sometimes accepting help was more problematic than continuing in the state of engulfment.

The balancing/boundary setting mode

The essence of this lies in having an element of separation between the carer and the situation. Carers in this category placed greater value on their own autonomy, and made space for their own interests. For some, the most important factor in allowing them to adopt this approach was their adjustment to the realities of their caring situation. For example, in relation to dementia, realizing that the person's odd and sometimes hurtful behaviour was not meaningful in any interpersonal way could be an important stage in adjustment, allowing them to move on towards a more limited, problem-solving approach. The neutrality in the meaning and cause of the disability is in contrast to the continuing guilt experienced by some carers who felt they were responsible for the disability and, as we have seen, were engulfed by that belief.

Some carers maintained their balancing mode by adopting a boundary setting approach. As we have seen, in Chapter 3, Mrs Todd used the physical arrangements of the house as a means of achieving psychic space for herself. Her boundary-setting extended to tasks of caring also. She got the district nursing service to give her husband a weekly enema because it was more then she wanted to do, and she commented: 'I think I do enough.' She criticized carers who allowed the cared-for person to bully them, and drawing on experiences from the multiple sclerosis group that her husband used to chair, commented: 'I think if you let them get the better of you, you've had it. You've got no life at all.' She described a woman who was always demanding help from her sister and would do nothing for herself: 'Well you see, I think that's how you let them get you down.' Mrs Todd was unusual in the degree to which she articulated the importance of maintaining her position in the relationship, of not being swamped by caring and of setting limits, but elements of this approach were shared by other carers.

Some carers were able to establish a balancing boundary setting mode as a result of adopting a self-identity as a carer. These carers had a clear picture of themselves as full-time carers who were of value to society and who deserved support in their chosen activity. Some made the point that they were saving the state considerable sums of money; this attitude carried over into their response to getting help from services. The clearest examples of this were both men, Mr Dilley and Mr Busby, who had come to interpret their caring as a form of occupation. Both were unemployed; the first through caring, the second not. There are parallels with Ungerson's study where she suggests that men adopt a language of occupation in their accounts of caring, and that that provides them with a technique with which to manage the caring and distance themselves from it (Ungerson 1987).

For some carers the shift towards regarding themselves self-consciously as a carer occurred under the influence of contact with voluntary organizations or carer support groups. These could be an important source of consciousness raising. Others appeared to have been affected by the general growth in public consciousness, reflected in TV, radio and magazine items, familiarizing people with the idea of being a 'carer'. Contact with service providers could also be a source of this self-perception as a carer. However, the reorientation was achieved, the effect was to reinforce the carers' own sense of worth and encourage them to articulate the importance of their activity.

Last, some carers in this category were able to be detached from the situation because they had a cool emotional relationship with the cared-for person. Their caring was characterized by the performance of certain tasks or exercise of certain responsibilities, but that was as far as it went. This appeared to be particularly associated with carers who looked after a sibling. One carer who was caring for a brain-damaged and behaviourally-difficult husband provides a slightly different example of this. She coped partly by using a boundary technique: he was confined to one downstairs room while the family ate and socialized in the other; but this was also partly because she no longer felt any love for him. This 'resolution' was not sufficiently total for her to escape all distress, and there was a sense in which her response was a mixed one that still contained elements of the engulfed mode. The case does illustrate, however, the ways in which emotional detachment, even coldness, can make caring easier. It is one of the ironies of caring that the emotional forces that draw you into it can also threaten your psychic survival and with it your capacity to continue caring.

If we ask for whom was this the dominant response, there appeared, not surprisingly, to be some relationship between time and mode of response. Some carers started in the engulfed mode but after a period of adjustment moved to a more balancing one. This pattern of movement was particularly characteristic where the disability was of sudden onset. Many of the parents of adults with learning difficulty had gone through a similar process of initial crisis and subsequent adjustment. Time did not always produce this transition; some carers' circumstances were such that they remained engulfed. The resolution represented by the balancing mode could be unstable, and carers were sometimes thrown back into an engulfed mode by some personal reversal, often with no link to caring.

We have already noted the association of the engulfed mode with gender, and the implications of this are carried through into the balancing mode. It appeared that more men than women found they could detach themselves in some degree from the situation. This did not necessarily mean they were unaffected by the experience, nor that some were on occasions distressed by it; however, they did seem better able to pull back and protect their sense of autonomy. This was particularly characteristic of male spouses caring for wives with dementia or severe physical problems. The objectively observable level of burden was also relevant, with some balancing carers able to adopt this mode because of their relatively light burden.

Carers who adopted this mode appeared to find it easier to accept help. Receiving assistance was not interpreted as a sign of personal failure. Those carers who adopted a pragmatic, matter-of-fact approach to caring were able to extend this into their relations with services, regarding them as a useful form of resource available to help them in their task of caring. For a small number, this mode of adjustment underwrote a more pro-active approach to services. This was most clearly detectable among those who had adopted a career model of caring: they were able to push service providers into action and to make demands both for themselves and the people they looked after. This help-seeking, pro-active approach was only adopted by a minority, and it would be quite wrong to see the balancing mode as resulting in a confident and assertive approach. The majority of carers remained passive in their relation to services; and it was more a question of accepting and perhaps negotiating with services than of actively seeking help.

The symbiotic mode

Here carers gain in a positive way from their role as a carer, to the extent indeed that they would not wish the responsibility and its consequences to be taken from them. The approach was most characteristic of parents caring for a child with learning disabilities or diagnosed as schizophrenic, particularly where one parent, often the mother, was left caring on her own. Mrs Harrison, as we have seen, relied on her son, who was diagnosed as schizophrenic, for company and help with her own declining health. She had made her life around caring for him and had no wish for him to leave. This response was found among a number of parents. Mr Coney, the father of a disabled daughter, rejected angrily all thoughts of his daughter living away from them, and remarked that having her with them in the future was one of the benefits of her disability.

Of course, most caring contains some aspects of benefit for the carer. People try to make the best of their lives, and this includes caring. Caring rests on intimate relationships, and most carers have feelings of love for their dependant, however mixed with other emotions. While not endorsing the view of those who assert that the manifestly obvious disbenefits must be being balanced by gains of some sort (Knapp 1984), we accept that there are often countervailing benefits. In using the term 'symbiotic', however, we are implying something that goes beyond such minor elements and encompasses situations where the carer derives positive benefits from their role, where they have no real wish for it to cease, and where their and the cared-for person's needs are mutually reinforcing. (We have excluded spouses from the category, for the reason that marriage can be seen as containing, of its nature, expectations of symbiosis; our aim here is to distinguish those cases where the symbiotic relationship arose in relation to the caring itself.)

As we have noted this is most often the response where the carer is a parent. It is also associated with situations where the physical burden of caring is not great, and, more important, where there are no serious behavioural problems. The main consequence of this mode for services was that carers were reasonably happy to accept service help so long as it did not threaten their own role as the carer. Services that improved the life of the cared-for person were welcome, but anything more extensive was not. Services aimed at relieving the carer were regarded as largely irrelevant.

There are important parallels between the three responses outlined here and those presented by Lewis and Meredith in their study of daughters caring for mothers. In this study 'balancing' carers balance the demands of caring with other work and family roles. They experience caring as stressful because it makes competing demands. By contrast, those whose caring is 'integrated' with the experiences of the their previous life, suffer no such conflict. These were usually single women who had always shared a household with their mother. They have similarities with the 'symbiotic' category described above, except that in Lewis and Meredith's account their relationships with their mothers are often problematic and stressful, whereas the essence of the symbiotic mode is that it causes few problems for the carer. Those carers whom Lewis and Meredith term 'immersed', saw caring as the focus of their lives. They were often, as were the 'engulfed', under the domination of their mothers (Lewis and Meredith 1988).

The responses described here, however, are refracted though a different and more varied set of relationships, and apply to both men and women; indeed, gender and relationship are both clearly significant in the different modes of response. The parallels are, however, striking, and suggest an objective coherence in the responses that carers adopt. A further set of parallels can be found in the literature on responses to chronic illness, where Herzlich (1973) distinguishes three responses: illness as destroyer, as occupation and as liberator. These link across to the engulfed, balancing and symbiotic modes.

The service provider's view

The attitude of the carer towards his or her caring role clearly affected how the service provider interpreted the situation. Service providers did not distinguish between the three modes of response directly, but were aware of the consequences of them. Service providers repeatedly emphasized that the carers who got help were those who were assertive and put themselves forward. In their view, this was the central truth about service delivery for carers. Because resources are insufficient, aims to some degree vague and unachievable, with few guidelines on priorities, service providers accept that who gets help is to some degree determined by factors extraneous to 'need'. Service providers did not in general seek out cases, and they responded only to those who came into their orbit and made themselves visible. This filtering of demand was not seen as ideal, but was recognized as a fact of life, structuring service response.

As we have seen, the balancing/boundary-setting carers tended to be more assertive and to have a stronger sense that they deserved help. Boundary-setting also enabled a carer to stop at certain points, and say that something was more than he or she was willing to do. The capacity to place limits was important in negotiations with service providers. Service providers often operate on the discretionary margin; they have limited resources and can only deploy them on occasions. They tend therefore to wait to see what response the carer will make. It is in the pauses of such exchanges that the capacity or otherwise of the carer to set limits or be assertive becomes important.

Sometimes service providers were themselves involved in encouraging carers to adopt a more assertive approach. Contact with services could sometimes introduce carers to the professional language of caring, and encourage them to see their circumstances in that framework rather than one simply of family obligation or love. Service providers sometimes tried to give permission to carers to accept help, to tell them in effect what was a legitimate expectation. This could be particularly important for engulfed carers who could in general see no such legitimacy. Some service providers, usually those with a social work background, also attempted to build up the self-esteem of carers in ways that would promote their sense of autonomy and with it their capacity to manage and limit their involvement. As we have seen, however, few carers came into extended contact with such practitioners. There were also limits as to how far service providers could pursue such approaches. Their professional values meant that many of them wanted to work with carers in this way, but the realities of available resources meant that they could not afford to do so. The approach tended to be applied selectively and, as we shall see, only in the context of certain relationships and age groups.

The attitude to carers who were assertive or who put themselves forward could, however, be ambivalent. In describing the attitudes of carers, service providers sometimes deployed a moral language in which there was a note of criticism. Because there was so little in the way of help available, no carer in the study received assistance that on an individual basis could be regarded as inappropriate, but service providers sometimes implied that certain carers, as a result of the attitude they adopted, got more help than they 'deserved'. Service providers, on occasions, drew a distinction between 'appropriate' help and help that was fully 'deserved', and this clearly had its roots in tensions around the negotiation of services in a context of chronic shortfall.

Sometimes service providers described the attitudes of carers in terms of their virtuousness or otherwise. Service providers used phrases like 'she's a real carer' or 'she could do more to help'; they described carers in terms of being a 'caring daughter' or a 'neglectful husband'. Virtuous carers featured more often than did neglectful ones, partly because the latter tended to be reclassified as 'family' and were no longer seen within a carer framework. These moral judgments affected practice in complex ways. Sometimes being virtuous meant in effect that you did not 'need' help, but sometimes it meant that you deserved a bit of compensatory support. Moral language about caring often arose in association with an unease felt by some service providers that they were unable in their practice to reflect values they felt were shared by everyone. In particular they felt that the priorities they had to operate meant that they sometimes 'rewarded' the neglectful by putting in extra help, or, more often, failed to reward the virtuous.

The role of the cared-for person

The negotiation of services cannot be understood without consideration of the role of the cared-for person. Not all exert a direct influence on decisions concerning service provision. Some are unable to do so by virtue of conditions like dementia; others adopt – or have forced upon them – a passive stance, going along with what is arranged by their carer. Some, however, are active, even dominant, participants. There are three main ways in which they exert an influence on service negotiation. First, the attitude adopted to their disability can be significant. Some underplayed their disability, asserting their competence in the face of the world.. Carers would often collude in this, helping them to hide their difficulties. As a result, however, the carer's role was sometimes underplayed or made invisible; service providers were often not aware of the full consequences of the disability for the carer. This hiding of disability behind a barrier of privacy was particularly characteristic of spouse carers.

Some disabled people exerted a more direct influence, refusing to accept certain forms of help. This applied in particular to respite – the idea of which was disliked, even feared, by many. Carers understandably responded to these feelings; in many cases the possibility of respite was never overtly raised, though the carer would have liked some form of break. Some refusals of help by the disabled person arose less from a rooted dislike of the service than from expectations embedded in the relationship. Some disabled people assumed that *only* the carer could or should look after them, and this excluded the possibility of any service help. This response was particularly characteristic of men being cared for by their wives.

Last, the disabled person could exert an influence through his or her ability to control the interaction between the carer and the service provider. At its most extreme the disabled person was able to exclude the carer from all contact with the service provider. This was particularly the case with medical consultations where, if the disabled person attended the hospital alone, the carer could remain literally invisible. There was no possibility of an exchange regarding their needs or perceptions, unless instigated directly by the cared-for person. This did happen on occasions, but it was rare. Disabled people were understandably reluctant to acknowledge in public that they were a source of burden or stress to their families.

Service providers respond to the presence of the cared-for person, endorsing the legitimacy of their influence in the process of negotiating services. First and foremost, this arises because the disabled person and not the carer is the client or patient. Their needs and interests occupy centre stage, and the legitimacy of their exerting control over service negotiation is accepted and at times actively promoted. Sometimes the legitimacy of their control was underwritten by the ways in which the service provider practised. As we have seen, hospital consultants, through their pattern of consultation, reinforced the ability of the disabled person to control the service interaction. The exclusion of the carer was not a conscious aim but arose as an unintended consequence. Sometimes, however, doctors excluded the carer intentionally, emphasizing the confidentiality of the doctor–patient relationship, and the consequent moral right of the cared-for person to exclude the carer from knowledge about his or her condition. This moral right, as we shall see shortly, operated differentially between conditions, depending on the 'moral status' of the cared-for person. Relationship also affects the legitimacy of sharing information, but to a lesser degree. Even marital relations do not necessarily override the general principle of confidentiality, and not all doctors would discuss a patient's condition with a spouse.

All service providers endorsed the right of the cared-for person to determine the nature of service provision. They varied, however, in the degree to which they were willing to compromise that right in the interest of the carer. The tendency to focus exclusively on the obligation to the disabled person was more characteristic of medical as opposed to social care professionals, though there was variation among doctors, with psychogeriatricians more willing to incorporate the wishes of the carer, and consultants of physical medicine focusing more exclusively on the patient.

The role of other kin

Kin play a part in the negotiation of services in two ways. The first is in their role as the surrounding social 'chorus', commenting on and judging the actions of the carer. Part of the carers' responses to service support arose from what they perceived to be the views of it held by their relatives. Kin have a particular importance in this, for caring is embedded in kinship obligation, and this gives special weight to the views of wider kin about the activities of the carer. A number of carers drew on the support of family members in their decisions to take certain steps or pursue certain forms of help. In general, the role of kin was presented as a positive one, giving permission to the carer to give more regard to him or herself and strengthening his or her resolve to pursue help, though there were instances when kin appeared to block the carer seeking help. The role of kin in giving permission was particularly important because of the way in which some carers had internalized a punishing account of their obligations. The wider social world was often presented as an exacting, potentially critical voice, and this was the case even where there had been no direct expression of criticism. As a result, carers often appeared to be in need of encouragement and permission to seek help. This was particularly relevant to those carers whose response was one of engulfment.

The second potential role of kin in the mediation of service receipt is as direct providers of care. We found, in line with other studies, that such involvement was limited (Sinclair 1990; Hills 1991). Caring largely devolved on an individual carer, and shared care was rare. Moreover, what the wider kin network did was circumscribed in character. Once again, this followed a pattern revealed in other work (Litwak and Kulis 1983); families helped with more distant and social aspects, such as sitting with the cared-for person, providing transport or shopping, and were rarely involved in the intimate tasks of personal care. Many carers were reluctant to ask for help from their families. As with Parker's study (1993) of younger couples, many older carers expressed reservations about turning to their children for help, emphasizing that they had their own lives to live. Carers thus put limits on the sorts and levels of help they would seek or accept from their families. From the carer's point of view, there was no simple model of substitution operating whereby they sought help first from family and, only when that had failed, from the formal sector. Carers did not necessarily regard formal services as a substitute for informal help, but a parallel and different source of help. Having a son or daughter in the area did not in their eyes mean that it was unnecessary or illegitimate to seek formal help.

Service providers were rarely in direct contact with the wider kin, but the assumptions they made about them could sometimes affect the negotiation and provision of services. Service providers appeared on occasions to take a different view of the issue of substitution from that of carers, or at least to operate according to different priorities. As we have seen, there were instances where the service providers had made a moral assumption that the wider family would help, with, for example, bathing when the carer was ill, without asking if this was in fact the case. As a result they did not provide service help to the carers, who felt pressurized into going to their families when they did not want to do so.

Normative expectations structuring caring

We now turn to a set of factors that operate at a more directly normative level, structuring expectations about caring and service receipt. They affect how the balance of authority and interest between the carer and the cared-for person is perceived; they also structure the expectations of both carers and service providers as to what are appropriate interventions in particular circumstances.

Relationship

Different relationships contain different normative expectations concerning caring. The obligations and expectations that spouses feel are different from those of children or other kin. It is clear that service providers to a large degree share these assumptions about the meaning of different relationships and that these have consequences for how they respond to the situation and the forms of help that they suggest and provide.

Spouse carers tend to see the support they give as a natural extension of the love and support that is a mutual expectation of contemporary marriage (Parker 1993). Nearly all forms of care-giving – except those of a technical, medical character – fall under this assumption. Marital relations are also regarded as defining an area of privacy. A number of spouse carers put a barrier around the relationship and regarded the involvement of the service provider as unwelcome. Service providers tended to share this concept of privacy and hold back from intruding in spouse relations. Marriage also includes an assumption that the couple will spend much of their free time together. This expectation which applies to 'normal' social life, made it difficult for spouse carers to articulate or even contemplate a wish for some time away from their partner. Service providers shared these expectations, and as a result often failed to perceive the strain imposed on some couples by constantly being together, or to respond to it by offering support that would allow the carer to create some time for him or herself.

Taken-for-granted assumptions about marriage, closeness and love could also blind service providers to problems, when they were otherwise sympathetic to the carer. An overemphasis on the tragic nature of caring and the heroic response of the carer could sometimes lead to a failure to perceive ways in which the carer's social and emotional life could be improved. This did not apply exclusively to spouse carers, but tended to be associated with that relationship. Being part of a couple could also affect the way service providers saw the transition to institutional care. This was far more likely to be seen as a negative outcome and a failure of the service system, than when the carer and cared-for person were not married. In general, this interpretation was one that was shared by the spouses. Service providers would go to much more extreme lengths to support the continuance of caring where it was between spouses, and at times this involved maintaining situations that were clearly on the brink of collapse.

Where the cared-for person is a parent, the assumptions are different. Privacy is less strongly defended, and there is a greater tradition of autonomy and separation. This is particularly the case where the household is not shared, or where co-residence has only been established after a long period of independence. The normative expectation of giving care also appears to be less absolute and more open to individual negotiation than is the case with spouse carers. The attitudes of service providers reflect these assumptions. Service providers, for example, tended to recognize the competing claims of carers' other family relationships, and regarded responding to these as legitimate. The transition into institutional care was also seen in a less negative fashion, and service providers were more willing to support, even at times to encourage, younger carers in the decision to give up caring for their parent.

Where the caring is of a parent for an adult child, the moral assumptions are again different. Caring is often seen by the parents – particularly where the condition is congenital – as an extension of the responsibilities of child care, and that model remains a powerful one structuring their expectations. That it requires the continuing 'childishness' of the cared-for person can lead to conflict between the carer and service providers. In these situations, the expectation of staying together is often more strongly held by the parents than by the service providers who would like to see the cared-for person moving on to independence. Parents often assume that they will remain responsible for the situation and in control of the main decisions concerning caring. Once again service providers may not regard this as legitimate, and may emphasize the autonomy of the cared-for person. These differences will be explored further in the next section.

Moral status

The 'moral status' of the cared-for person is constructed by the interaction of two elements: mental competence and achieved adulthood. 'Mental competence' relates to the cognitive ability of the cared-for person and can be impaired in various ways: accidental brain damage, severe mental illness and dementia in old age. 'Achieved adulthood' refers to the degree to which an individual has established an independent adult life. This usually involves such markers as earning a living, having a private sexual life, living away from home, owning property, marriage and parenthood. Taken together these profoundly affect the assumptions that are made concerning the role of the carer.

Different client groups can be placed according to these two axes (Figure 3). A physically disabled adult where the onset of the problem occurred in middle or later years, as with multiple sclerosis or chronic heart problems, is represented by point PD. Here the person has experienced a fully independent adult life and there is no mental impairment. In the case of a physically disabled adult where the origin of the disability was congenital (CD), though mental competence may not be impaired, full adulthood in the eyes of the world is less easily achieved, particularly where the person has not left home. They are thus seen as high on mental competence, but low on achieved adulthood.

An elderly mentally infirm person, by contrast, is no longer mentally competent, but has lived a long life in which he or she has established an independent social identity. They are likely to have married and may own

Figure 3 Moral status

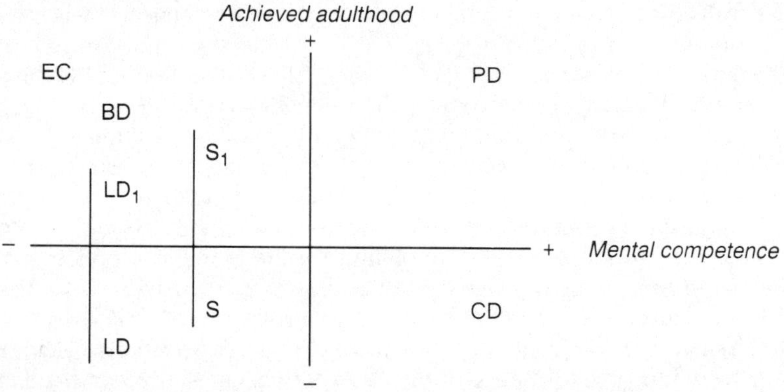

property. He or she is high on achieved adulthood, but low on mental competence, and is represented by point EC. A young adult diagnosed as schizophrenic has experienced some impairment of his/her mental faculties. Prior to the first episode of the illness, however, he or she was firmly on a trajectory that would lead to independent adulthood. The onset of the illness however disrupts those expectations. Where that occurred prior to marriage or leaving home, the degree of achieved adulthood is limited (point S). Where it occurs later, possibly after marriage, the adulthood is not so compromised.

In the case of someone with a learning disability, their mental competence is in some degree limited, and so is their achieved adulthood (point LD). Unlike the adult with mental health problems, they have not had an earlier passage in their life when the assumption was that they would achieve full adult status. This contrasts with the situation of a brain-damaged adult (BD) where their mental ability may be very similar to that of someone with learning disabilities, but where having lived as an independent adult, working, owning a house, perhaps marrying, they have achieved an independent social identity.

Good practice in the fields of learning disabilities and mental health aims to counter these tendencies and encourage clients or patients towards assuming an independent adult persona. Progressive practitioners therefore place these individuals at points S_1 and LD_1. From the point of view of most parent carers, however, their position is still at S and LD. This difference of perspective over moral status is a major source of conflict between parent-carers and certain service providers. With older people, the judgments tend to be less divergent, and carers and service providers more inclined to share the same perceptions.

It is clear that the dimension of moral status, particularly taken in conjunction with relationship, has a significant effect on the way in which society views the moral and quasi-legal relationship between the carer and the cared-for person. How far is the cared-for person to be regarded as autonomous? Does the carer have rights to be consulted or to exercise their preferences in the situation? These questions have consequences for the negotiation of services, affecting the attitude of both carers and service providers. Who makes decisions and on whose behalf? How far should the cared-for person exercise control over services and over whether he or she uses them? What rights does the carer have? Can the carer insist on help? Can he or she exercise control over the cared-for person for their own good? How far can they do this in their own interests? All these questions are affected by the perceived moral status of the cared-for person.

Time and the future

The third of the normative factors framing the relationship between the carer and the cared-for person is that of time. Caring takes place within a time trajectory, but it is one that involves two people. How the future is constructed depends upon the degree to which these two trajectories overlap; this in turn affects the meaning given to the current situation and the role that service providers play in it. The difference between the generations is of central importance here, and carers can be divided into three groups accordingly. The first group are the parents of disabled offspring whether the disability is physical or mental. In these cases, carers can normally expect that their children will survive them. The future therefore involves a separate life for the disabled person. The second group are of the same generation. Most of these carers are spouses. Here there is no reason to assume that either the cared-for person or the carer will die first; the presence of disability in many cases does not necessarily predict an earlier death. The third group are those of the younger generation, mainly offspring. Here there is an assumption that the older person will die before the carer. What is at issue is the passage through that period of caring when the carer's life is often in a state of abeyance, with employment or social life postponed for an indefinite period.

The crucial distinction is between the first group, where the cared-for person can usually be expected to survive the carer, and the second and third groups, where this is not the case. Knowing that the cared-for person will have a future beyond present caring clearly affects the attitudes of both carers and service providers. Parents often lack confidence in the continuation of service support. Their career as carers has meant that they have seen many service providers come and go. They can be sceptical of the promises of agencies, and fearful of future cuts in service. They are often reluctant to trust public agencies, and cynical of their capacity to deliver the independent living that normalization theory leads service providers to emphasize. As a result, many carers assert alternative, less independent, goals for their offspring. Some carers attempt to secure the future through the use of money or other resources, but this is itself uncertain, and not open to all. Service providers are similarly conscious of the existence of an independent future, and their judgments in the present are affected by that eventuality. They may press for respite in a hostel not simply to give the parents a break, but also as a means towards a separate future.

Social structural factors

The normative factors outlined above relate quite closely to the nature of caring. We now turn to a set of factors that operate at a more general, social structural level. They still affect expectations concerning the appropriate service response, but do so as part of their more pervasive influence within society.

Gender

As we noted in Chapter 1, there is a growing body of work over the past decade that has explored the links between caring and gender (Finch and Groves 1983; Graham 1983; Land and Rose 1985; Ungerson 1987, 1991; Dalley 1988; Lewis and Meredith 1988; Baldwin and Twigg 1991). Much of the earlier work was concerned with the differential burden of caring borne by men and women, although the perception of this has been modified by the evidence from the *General Household Survey* (*GHS*) suggesting that more men are involved in caring than was previously understood, albeit at a lesser level of intensity and most commonly in spouse relations (Green 1988; Parker 1993). But work on gender and caring has also had a wider significance, exploring how caring is seen to be 'natural' for women, and linked to other aspects of the female role, both at home and in the world of work. Gender itself mediates the experience of caring, affecting how carers interpret their situations and the potential role of services in them.

Graham (1991) argues that the feminist emphasis on gender as *the* explanatory variable in informal care needs to be modified, in particular by a recognition of the importance of other factors such as class and race. In our study, gender was not treated as an independent variable, but as one that was itself mediated through the responses of carers to their caring role. Thus the engulfed response was more characteristic of female carers, and the balancing/boundary-setting approach more characteristic of males. Men appear to find it easier to separate themselves from the caring situation, to set limits on their involvement and to see themselves as 'professional carers' who should legitimately receive support. Women, by contrast, were more likely to subordinate their interest to those of the person they looked after, to be less detached, and to regard the acceptance of help as a sign of failure. This pattern reflects other findings concerning the greater instrumentality of men, the tendency we have already referred to for them to see moral questions in terms of rules rather than relationships, and the impact on their attitudes of involvement with the world of work. The association of gender with mode of response was not an absolute one, and was mediated by other personal and cultural factors.

If we turn to the attitudes of service providers, there was some evidence that gender operates as a mediating factor on practice. One of the ways in which gender assumptions were significant was in relation to the visibility of the carer. Actions that were noteworthy in a male carer and resulted in him being recognized as such, were passed over when performed by a female, subsumed under her general domestic role. This response seemed particularly common among GPs, who were less exposed to professional values stressing antisexism and whose practice in relation to carers drew more heavily on their personal values and experiences than was the case with, for example, social workers. For similar reasons the notion of the 'virtuous carer' was also affected by gender. To be regarded as virtuous, a male carer needed to undertake less care because service practitioners had lower expectations of the help likely to be provided by men.

In general service providers asserted that gender had – and should have – no relevance to the provision of help, though occasionally a respondent would add that they felt it was probably the case that female carers got less assistance. This was never, however, described as something that arose in their own practice. There was some evidence in the study, echoing work by Arber and her colleagues (1988) indicating that community nursing support was more commonly provided to male as opposed to female carers, although we had no clear evidence indicating whether the assumptions underlying this possible pattern were those of the carers or of the nurses. The one area where gender was – or had been – explicitly linked to allocation was in the home help service. Home help relates to a sphere of activity – domestic labour – that is heavily gendered. There has been a tradition in the service of treating male and female carers differently, with domestic help to elderly people being withheld where there was a female relative in the locality, but not where there was a male. These traditions as we saw in Chapter 4 were now regarded, by managers at least, as obsolete, though there was evidence of their survival at the level of front-line personnel.

Age

Age is a major factor structuring people's expectations for and perceptions of themselves, although a distinction needs to be drawn between chronological age and stage in the life cycle or life course (Harris 1987). Carers held different expectations about their lives depending on their age. These expectations did not necessarily relate directly to caring, but did influence the way in which caring was seen to have affected their lives. Some elderly carers did not expect to go out socially, and saw the restriction imposed by caring as little different from the other limitations of old age. As a result they made no attempt to get help. This view was not, however, shared by all older carers, and some still wanted a chance to go out and enjoy themselves.

Some younger carers believed that service providers discriminated against them, and that support was biased in favour of elderly carers. This view was expressed particularly in relation to respite and day care for people with dementia. There was some indication that service providers did indeed regard being old and a carer as a double burden, but it was not possible to say how far this reflected additional factors such as relationship. Sometimes a service provider appeared to operate a reverse discrimination based, not on implicit assumptions about stress and the difficulties of being both old and a carer, but on assumptions concerning normal life. Service providers reacted differently to carers who were in their twenties from those in their fifties. Helping young carers to develop a life for themselves, to work and perhaps to marry, was seen as a legitimate aim for service support. For middle-aged carers, however, these aims were not given the same emphasis. As one young assistant social worker put it, carers in their fifties accept that 'their days are gone'. In such cases he would give support 'as required . . . [but] would be careful not to overstep the mark'.

Social class and race

The scope of the study did not allow for any systematic treatment of issues of class or race. An account of the structural factors mediating the carer's relationship with services would, however, be incomplete without reference to them. Since social class is an important variable in determining people's experience of disability and ill health (Blaxter and Pearson 1982), it is reasonable to assume that it is of importance in structuring people's experience of informal care. Middle-class carers are likely to have greater access to resources both in the sense of material surroundings and money with which to purchase care (Parker 1990a). The impact of caring on employment also varies according to class, with carers in manual jobs much more likely to have to give up their work (Baldwin 1985). Social class is also an important variable in considering the response of service providers. Middle-class people are more aware of service provision, and their social skills and power of articulation mean that they are more likely to become visible to a service provider and to have a productive interaction than their working-class counterparts (Mayer and Timms 1970; Stimson and Webb 1975; Robinson 1978; Buckquet and Curtis 1986; Ungerson 1987; Rojek *et al.* 1988; Robinson and Stalker 1992). We should assume that social class is relevant in the negotiation of services for carers also.

Race raises similar issues to social class. As we have noted, Graham (1991) has argued that recent feminist conceptualizations of caring have failed to incorporate dimensions of race and class, and as a result have limited our understanding to gender issues only. A similar critique has been put forward by Williams (1989) in the context of social policy more widely. The importance of race in structuring a person's experience of the world has been well established (Kiple and King 1981; Pearson 1983; Norman 1985; Donovan 1986). Work on informal care and service provision has tended to ignore black people and has focused almost exclusively on the white population of the United Kingdom. Work on services has established the unsuitable and inaccessible nature of much service provision for black communities (Holland and Lewando-Hundt 1987; Connelly 1988; Atkin and Rollings 1993). Black people are often disadvantaged in their contact with service provision as a result of racism (Rooney 1987). The ways in which service provision is organized and delivered in relation to people who form black minorities have also been identified as an important factor in understanding this (Atkin 1991).

Chapter 10 STRUCTURING

In Chapter 9 we looked at factors mediating the relationship between carers and service provision, concentrating on features of the individual carer or cared-for person, and noting that assumptions relating to these affected not just the judgments of service providers but also those of carers and the people for whom they care. We now turn to a different set of factors structuring the responses of service providers. These relate to the organizational and professional contexts within which service providers operate. Our focus in this book has largely been on individual service providers. This has partly been a product of the methodology employed in the study on which this book draws; but it fits also with the theoretical emphasis in our work on the front-line worker and on the analysis of services at this level. This emphasis was discussed in greater detail in Chapter 2 in relation to the work of Lipsky.

We recognize, however, that service providers operate in a wider organizational context. In this chapter we explore the role of professional and institutional factors in structuring the responses of service providers in ways that affect how far and in what ways they incorporate carers into their practice. The factors we concentrate upon are all relatively local to the situation we discuss. They are about the particular consequences for carers of patterns of practice or of organization. They are not, by and large, about the larger organizational and political context provided by, for example, the National Health Service or personal social services or the welfare state. These are important structuring contexts, but they are not the focus of this chapter.

The first of our structuring factors relates to the distinction between medical and social care. The traditional focus of medicine is on the patient. Medicine defines the problem first in terms of physiological phenomena – the condition or the malfunctioning organ or subsystem; the second in terms of the individual patient – his or her body. It plays down wider aspects of the patient's emotional, material and social existence. That is not to say, of course, that the recognition of the significance of these aspects – particularly the emotional – is not part of medical practice and has been so over the centuries. It is, however, a subordinated part, a minor tradition, particularly in the context of the rise of scientific- and technologically-based medicine. The narrowness of the medical account, as well as its authoritarianism, has been subject to much criticism from the disability lobby who have argued that the primary 'problems' of disabled people lie in the difficulties of daily living and the limitations imposed on them by a disablist society and not in any medical condition that they might have (Oliver 1990). Escape from medical dominance, both in the sense of the interpretation imposed and the control exercised by service personnel, has been an important element in the struggle for independent living; that struggle has been carried across into debates about normalization for people with learning disabilities.

A social care focus, by contrast, starts from the wider context of the client. Its focus is on social, as opposed to physiological, functioning, and it draws on a different knowledge base, that of sociology, social psychology and the related theories that underpin the psychotherapeutic tradition. The wider material, social and interpersonal aspects of the client's situation are seen as central to the understanding and definition of their problems as well as to effective intervention. Although the focus is still predominantly on the individual client, it is often widened to include, particularly under the influence of family systems theory, the family as a whole. These tendencies are strongest, of course, in the field of child care, but their influence carries over into social services more generally.

This broad distinction between the medical and the social care traditions has major implications for carers. Blaxter showed in the 1970s how a disabled person's contact with the service system influenced the manner in which they perceived and defined their own disability (Blaxter 1976). Medical services emphasize the medical aspects, while social services emphasize the social, and this is carried over into the responses of disabled people. Carers experience a similar process of definition, although in their case the defining force is not services in relation to their own disability but the disability of the person they care for. People with physical disability or chronic illness were more likely to be in contact with medical services; that fact affected how the situation of their carers was perceived. Those caring for someone with learning disability were more likely – at least in recent years – to be in contact with social services. Again that produced a different set of service assumptions in relation to the carer.

The initial point of contact can also be significant in determining into which service ambit the carer will fall. Most carers have little experience of the service system and do not know how to obtain help. They often contact the most accessible service provider. Who that person is can determine how the problem is defined and the subsequent pathways into help they may be sent along, since there is a tendency for service providers to have greater knowledge of and confidence in their own service sector, and to restrict their referrals within it.

As we have seen, helping carers is not regarded as a central aspect of medical practice. Carers drawn into this context tended to be seen as 'family' or 'relatives' – people who were ancillary to the patient, part of the background but not within the remit of practice. In so far as medical practitioners did perceive them as carers it was with an instrumental focus. Medicine is not, of course, monolithic and there are, as we have seen, systematic variations in the responses of clinicians. Geriatricians and psychogeriatricians were more likely to employ a social-care perspective within their work and to incorporate the needs of carers to some degree. Psychiatrists also recognized the significance of the emotional and familial circumstances of the patient, though their practice remained focused on the individual patient. Practitioners who worked within a social-care model did incorporate carers into their practice to a greater degree, though the difference should not be exaggerated. Although service providers who worked within a social care context had a clearer conception of carers and their needs, their dominant response was still an instrumental one. Carers were more visible to them than was the case with, for example, hospital consultants to whom they scarcely existed in professional terms, but it was a form of visibility that still made them secondary to the needs of the person for whom they cared.

The material/spatial context can also affect the way service providers work, exercising a powerful influence on the literal viability or otherwise of the carer. As we have seen, hospital doctors, and to some extent GPs, see patients in the context of the consulting room, and this imposes limitations on their knowledge of the carer and his or her circumstances. In this way a literal invisibility can reinforce a professional one. A similar process can occur in relation to day care where the boundaries of the day centre, its very walls, can limit the awareness of the carer. Most day-care staff do not work beyond the boundaries of the centre and they rely for their knowledge of carers on their willingness to put themselves forward and come into the centre. Their view of the situation is circumscribed by the boundaries of the building. Service providers whose practice is not spatially confined and who go into the home are, by contrast, more likely to be aware of the existence of a carer and of their circumstances. Thus home helps or staff providing aids may be in a better position to assess the circumstances of a carer, although the narrower remit of their work means that they are less likely to operate on the basis of that knowledge. Those GPs who did call at the home often found a situation of which they were unaware.

Service providers are embedded within service traditions. These define the kinds of things they do and the sorts of services they are able to deploy. Services are legitimated by what they have traditionally done rather than what they aim to achieve. It is, for example, more plausible to describe the meals-on-wheels service in terms of providing a hot meal for a large number of elderly people in a kindly manner that draws on the traditions of the WRVS, as it is to talk about nutritional goals or community care outcomes. As we noted, however, in Chapter 2, policy interventions in relation to carers are not well defined. There is little in the way of a service tradition. Carers have come late on the scene in service terms, and have to fit into the way services have developed historically. Service providers have a limited range of things they can offer. As we noted in relation to social work, there is little evidence as yet of the deployment of complex or flexible packages of care. Most responses consist in a restricted range of off-the-peg interventions. Services are limited in what problems they address, and the 'problems' are themselves defined in large measure in terms of service solutions. As a result it is very important for the carer, if she or he is to obtain help, to have a problem that is service shaped, or at least that can be recast in that form. Carers, if they are to get help, have to fit into services that already exist.

Certain problems faced by carers were relatively difficult for service providers to address directly. This was particularly true of behavioural difficulties. Partly, this was because no totally effective intervention in this area existed: behavioural modification, drugs, counselling, respite could all play a part, but none wholly resolved the situation which carers often experienced as very stressful. Partly the problem, however, was that behavioural difficulties did not fit very clearly into any service or indeed into the remit of any one service provider. In short, they were not service-shaped.

Service providers found it much easier to respond where the difficulties could be fitted into a standard service response, and ideally where there were clear and defined tasks to perform, like household cleaning. This was all the more so where models of public and commercial provision already existed, as with domestic labour, laundry and catering. It is in the nature of personal care tasks, as we noted in Chapter 3, that they cannot be accumulated, and this poses problems of service delivery. Less clearly-focused anxieties that arose from the sense of 'being responsible' for the cared-for person were also harder to address. The chief exception to this pattern was where a 'service' had been modelled specifically on the activities of the carer and could thus offer a perfect substitution. Flexible care attendants schemes where the worker performs exactly the same tasks as the carer, often under her or his direction, are the clearest example of this and represent the conscious opposite of the principle of having to have a problem that is service-shaped.

Service providers at the front line typically operate in conditions of resource scarcity. This inevitably puts pressure on them and threatens their sense of themselves as professionals. One way in which they manage this tension, as we saw with district nurses, is by operating an in-or-out system that allows them to protect good practice by limiting its applications only to certain cases. Certain activities are identified as key and their performance constitutes a focal intervention around which other forms of help may be marshalled. In relation to district nurses the key activities are technical/medical ones. The existence of a focal intervention was the crucial factor in determining whether or not a carer would receive support from a nurse: responding to the needs of carers was present within the professional ideology, but was only activated in the presence of a focal intervention. In a similar way, although social workers supported carers by talking with them and allowing them to express their feelings, and this was seen as an appropriate part of their work, the route to such help was usually through assessment for some more concrete service like day care. Here the core of the response was defined less by the professional ideology than by the realities of social work practice with older and disabled people which is quite narrowly focused on providing practical help.

As important as having a focal intervention, was being in contact with a focal institution. Again we have noted how certain day hospitals, particularly for people with dementia, or day centres for people with learning disabilities operate as a focus for a range of services. The core activity may be day care or respite, but for those carers who are linked into it through the attendance of their relative, the institution potentially offers a wider network of support. There may be a carers' group; sometimes there are outreach workers in the form of attached CPNs or social workers, or direct links into the mental handicap team. In this case the needs of carers are more likely to be recognized and acted upon. Focal institutions also offer a form of support that continues over time. This brings us to the next distinction which is between services that are continuing as opposed to one-off.

'One-off' services are when a service provider makes an assessment, responds and then withdraws. Staff providing aids typically operate on this basis. To a significant degree GPs do also, with each consultation representing a discrete episode. 'Continuing' services, by contrast, remain in touch. Examples of continuing services are day centres, certain respite facilities that offer recurring relief and some mental handicap teams that keep clients more or less permanently on the books. Here service contact continues over time, sometimes long periods of time. Where services are continuing they are much better placed to monitor any changes in the circumstances of the carer and act upon them. They are also more effective in persuading sometimes reluctant carers to accept help. As we have noted, the negotiation of services, like respite, is important and may need to be undertaken slowly, building on confidence gained through more day-to-day contacts. One-off services that require carers to re-refer themselves pose an additional barrier. Carers as we noted are often diffident about putting themselves and their needs forward and they often lack knowledge of what is available and appropriate. Although GPs largely operate on a one-off basis, with the carer having to refer themselves each time, they do also represent a continuing point of contact. Carers feel that they have a GP, even though they may be different about approaching him or her. With social work, by contrast, as we have noted, the pattern of resolution and case closure was little understood or appreciated by carers who experienced their problems as continuing ones and expected services to reflect that fact.

Practitioners also vary in the degree to which they are reactive or proactive. Hunter and his colleagues (1988) suggested three types of response to carers: first, the proactive in which the service provider would identify unmet need and act on it as a matter of course, without being asked to do so by the carer; second, the reactive where the service provider only responded to the carer's requests, with the carer having to ask for help directly; third, that of floating, where the service provider moved between reactive and proactive. The response adopted depended on individual circumstances and resources available. The nature and organization of service provision, with a lack of resources and limits on time, often encouraged service providers to be reactive, even where their own professional values led them to subscribe to a more proactive model. As we have seen, occupational therapists in one of the areas were told to concentrate only on 'referred need' and discouraged from identifying further needs. General practitioners complained they could not respond to carers' needs because they did not have the time: the patient had to come first. Although social workers attempted to be proactive, they often found it difficult to maintain this approach because of the pressures of work. In general, carers expected service providers to be more proactive than they were. They assumed that once they had been in contact with a service providers like the GP or social worker they would have been informed of all the help that is available. They did not expect to have to push for such information and were angry if they subsequently discovered that help existed that they had not been told about.

Last, how the service provider defined his or her role in relation to other services could be important, in that this defines where they see their role ending and another's beginning. Consultants, for example, felt social issues should be dealt with by general practitioners. Day centres expected social workers to provide advice on benefits. These beliefs defined the limits of their role, and the help they would offer to the carer. The service provider's perception, knowledge and awareness of other service provision was an important factor in relation to onward referral. If a service provider had little knowledge of other forms of service provision, the carer would not be referred on. General practitioners often had little understanding of social services and little confidence in them. Social workers were similarly critical of GPs, and found it difficult to involve them in their cases.

Chapter 11 CARERS IN THE POLICY ARENA

At the start of this book we described how caring emerged as an academic and policy issue, achieving by the 1990s a position of self-conscious articulation. The study of carers and services has become a subject in itself. The time has now come to re-integrate that account of caring back into wider debates concerning social care. It is no longer possible or advisable to pursue the subject of support for carers in isolation from issues concerning the service system generally. There are four levels at which this integration needs to take place.

First there is the scope of the subject. As we saw in Chapter 2, carers are – potentially at least – pervasive within the service system. 'Services' for carers are not a distinct category, but are better understood in terms of the response of the service system as a whole to the carer issue. The service providers whose practice we analysed in Chapters 4 to 6 would not primarily think of themselves as acting for carers, and indeed as we saw some did not think in those terms at all.

Second, carers' views of services cannot be taken in isolation. Much of the earlier qualitative work on carers and services concentrated on eliciting carers' views about various forms of support. This was valuable, and the approach has informed our own work. But such accounts, in the absence of a parallel narrative from the service provider side, stand in isolation – comments made into a void and not placed in the context of the aims, purposes, tensions and constraints of service provision. In the chapters exploring the responses of service providers we have attempted to provide such a context.

Third, the needs and interests of carers have to be balanced against those of the cared-for person. As we have noted in Chapter 1, caring takes place in a relationship and this imposes an essential duality on the policy or academic analysis.

Fourth, support for carers has to be set within the context of debates concerning community care. The service questions presented by carers are not fundamentally different from those posed by other client groups. The issues are sometimes in a more complex form, but they are general to social welfare; there are direct parallels between how carers' needs and interests might be incorporated into the service system and how those of clients might be also.

Other work (Twigg 1993) has explored in more speculative form the mechanisms that might be employed to integrate carers into service delivery.

Here we concentrate on a more empirical discussion. How do carers fit within service provision? How might their needs and interests be incorporated into the new community care, and what can we learn from our study that is germane to the questions of case management, targeting, discretion and transparency? Before discussing these, we need to return to the issue of resources.

Limited resources and hard choices

Most of the literature on caring has avoided the question of resources. Work of a campaigning character does so naturally: its role is to highlight the issue and force the interests of carers onto the policy agenda. But the absence of discussion of resources extends also to the academic literature, much of which has remained at the stage of asserting the significance of carers and the 'costs' they bear but without attempting to balance them against those of others within the policy arena. Our study did not attempt to cost the various forms of support carers did or did not receive, and indeed as we argued in Chapter 2 the units of service approach that underlies costing methodologies is not one that reflects well the complex ways in which the service system responds to carers. Resource questions do, however, need to be addressed.

The claim has often been made that much can done for carers without significant additional resources. Evidence from our study suggests that this is in part true. It was certainly the case that service providers could be made more sensitive to the needs and interests of carers and that the resource implications of this were not great. What many carers wanted was recognition, advice, validation of their worth and a chance to talk, rather than major service inputs. They wanted their concerns listened to and their views consulted. Often it was the *way* in which the service was delivered rather than the amount that was the problem. Respite provides a good example of this, and we have noted the importance of the careful negotiation of the service, sensitive handling of the transitions in and out of care, and the systematic transmission of information about the cared-for person. These are all practice issues that can be addressed without great resource consequences.

Some of the ways of altering provision to meet the wishes of carers, however, have more significant costs attached to them. For example, as we have seen, there is a direct conflict between maximizing bed occupancy and providing the kind of flexible service that some carers want. If you are running a 'tuck-in' service it is, as we saw from the comments of the nursing manager, difficult to avoid putting some people to bed at an extremely early hour. Transport to day care illustrated some of the same tensions. What carers wanted, and felt was reasonable, was reliable transport that collected and returned the cared-for person at a stated time, preferably one that fitted their own activities. But this was often in direct conflict with the demands of organizing an efficient collection round, particularly in the context of uncertain traffic. It may be possible to make changes on the margins to improve the responsiveness of these services, but major alterations in their pattern would require additional resources.

Similar questions arise in relation to visibility. We have seen how the invisibility of carers – literal and metaphorical – can be a barrier to their being incorporated in service provision. We noted how service providers often failed to perceive the restrictedness suffered by spouse carers. A narrowly sectoral service focus, or an extreme emphasis on the patient, similarly created blind spots in service provision. The fact that many service providers never met the carer, or did so only in the company of the cared-for person, could also lead to a failure to appreciate the carer's needs. Once again, these are issues of practice that can be met by education and training rather than major service inputs. But making carers visible may itself have consequences for resources if service providers do more than simply recognize carers and incorporate them in decision-making. Not all needs can be met by greater sensitivity and awareness. Sometimes carers simply need services.

More services implies either additional resources or the retargeting of existing ones. This may mean retargeting standard services in the direction of carers. We have described the ways in which carers receive help from services that are currently aimed primarily at the cared-for person. We have also noted how services that have a potential role in supporting carers, such as the community nursing service, rarely fulfil it to any great extent: their priorities are elsewhere. Moves have begun, certainly in the home-care service, towards the explicit inclusion of carers' needs in decisions about allocation. But the reality of such developments is that they have taken place within a context of stable and sometimes reducing resources. Nationally, the home-care service has been under increasing pressure, to the extent that in some places it has effectively been withdrawn from all but the most frail. Retargeting mainstream services towards carers without a new injection of resources means withdrawing support from other clients. This is clearly contentious.

It is worth reiterating at this point that we had no evidence in the study of 'overprovision'. We had individuals who received more help than others in comparable situations, but this was never at a level that could be regarded as excessive. Although service providers, as we have seen, sometimes commented unfavourably on these carers, they never saw the help they received as inappropriate. There was no evidence therefore of extensive slack or misdirection of resources that would allow for carers' needs to be met within the same level of resources.

We did have clear evidence of shortfalls in the sense of services that carers would have valued and that would have materially improved their lives. Furthermore, there were important services that were unavailable in our two areas – Crossroads Care being an example – and for reasons of limited resources. Helping carers does therefore have resource implications. How great these are cannot be resolved simply by research. Ultimately, it is a quesion of how far society is willing to go in recognizing such needs. Claims for the cost-effectiveness of supporting carers have often been advanced, but never wholly established. The relationship is clearly present, but probably not as straightforwardly as is claimed. It is also of course not the only justification for supporting carers. Carers can legitimately make claims for support and relief in their own right.

The debate on community care

We now turn to a set of interconnected debates relating to community care. These turn around questions of needs and targets, discretion and specificity, flexibility and transparency. The entry point is case management.

Case management

Case management was developed in the United States as a means of overcoming the fragmentation and dislocation in a system that is project-based, relies on multiple funding and lacks a coherent organizational focus. It was brought to the UK in experimental form in the 1980s, particularly associated with the Kent Community Care Project (Challis and Davies 1986; Davies and Challis 1986). The approach was taken up and developed more widely in other experimental schemes (Dant and Gearing 1990; Richardson and Higgins 1992), and it now forms the chief plank in the new community care ushered in by the NHS and Community Care Act 1990 and the associated practice guidance, where it is termed care management (DH 1990). Claims have been made for its ability to deliver more flexible and closely tailored services in a way that maximizes their cost-effectiveness.

It is important to emphasize that case managers are in the same position in regard to carers as social workers and other professionals have been in the past. The issue remains the same: how far and in what way is the carer's interest incorporated into the assessment. In a similar way the potential conflict of interest between the carer and the cared-for person cannot be evaded. There is clearly no sense in having a separate case manager for each party, and case managers thus face the same difficulties in balancing the two interests as service providers do currently. The tensions and dilemmas of practice remain the same, except that in case management systems there is a tendency for them to be more focused and for policy aims to be made more explicit. Case management provides a structure for negotiation, but not the valuations that are fed into the negotiation. Just as case management can be run on high budget levels or on low ones, so too can it be run in regard of carers or in neglect of them. If in the definition of valued outcomes of the service, the well-being of carers *per se* rather than just the continuance of their caring, is regarded as a goal, case management will provide an important means of supporting carers. But there is no necessity for this. It is not part of the logic of the approach. Case management is of itself carer-neutral.

Concern has sometimes been expressed at the likely tendency for case management systems to adopt a residualist approach to carers (Parker 1990b). Maximizing the effectiveness of budgets is bound to produce a tendency to regard carers as a form of 'free good' whose input can be assumed. But in this, case management is doing no more than carrying forward, albeit in sharper form, the older tradition of seeing carers as a form of resource. Case management may make the incentive system more overt and underline it with budgetary responsibilities, but the essential logic is no different. The key question remains one of developing policy formulations in which the needs of carers are specifically included among the valued outcomes of the service.

Beyond this, what can we say from the research that is germane to the issue of case management? It is clear from the study that there will be many carers who will not come into the orbit of a case-management system. Case management itself in the full sense is likely to be available only on a limited basis; and many carers, as we have seen, are not linked into pathways that will lead them to such a service. We noted this in particular in relation to the carers of people with chronic physical illness or disability who are largely cared for in the medical sector. How far carers are visible to service providers and how far, and whether, they are incorporated into their practice depends on the professional background of the service provider: their training, their professional ideology, the culture of their job. Much thus turns on who is the case manager; claims for this role have been advanced by a variety of practitioners. As we have seen in the study, social workers were the most alert to the carer issue incorporating them to a greater degree in the assessment, though we noted that this did not necessarily lead to their receiving extensive support. GPs by contrast were more variable and *ad hoc* in their responses. Carers were rarely incorporated into their practice; many remained invisible to the doctor. GPs had little or no training in these social areas, and they tended to apply common-sense assumptions from their own social worlds. It was not that these made them unsympathetic to carers, but that it led them to apply rather stereotypical ideas about, for example, the role of women, or the 'virtuous' character of certain carers, and these meant that they did not go on to explore the ways in which the carer's situation could be alleviated. Some community nurses did have a perception of themselves as key workers or case managers, and they did recognize carers' needs, but they only acted upon them in the context of some form of acute medical intervention. Home-help organizers, by contrast, had a more limited view, one constrained by the remit of their role and by their lack of training. It is thus clear that the situation of carers will be affected by the professional background of the case manager; the incorporation of carers more extensive if the case manager is either a social worker or trained in the social care tradition, rather than a GP or other medically trained person.

Targeting

The key to successful case management lies in greater specificity of aims. One of the stumbling blocks to developing a more effective response to carers has been the absence of clear aims or targets for provision. We can explore the issues raised by this by looking at the target models that service providers currently do or do not implicitly employ.

It was clear that none of the service providers in the study operated a thoroughgoing *turning point system*, focusing resources exclusively on those who were 'on the brink' where there was a strong possibility of the carer collapsing or withdrawing care. This would represent an extreme version of the instrumental argument whereby support for carers is seen only in terms of support for disabled people and there is little concern for the needs of carers *per se*. Carers, as we have seen, sometimes believed that service providers did adopt this approach, requiring them to be on the brink of collapse before they would respond, but our evidence from the sample and from talking to service providers did not suggest that this was in fact the case. Service providers certainly did not operate on such a basis in any thoroughgoing or systematic way. The principal barriers to their doing so were the professional values they held, though these were also strengthened by values drawn from ordinary life. These value systems did not endorse such an approach. Targeting only on those about to give up was regarded as too openly exploitative to be acceptable in a social care context. Where service providers perceived the system as tending in such a direction, they regretted it.

Service providers also rejected the approach because of its implications for prevention. If one targets solely on individuals who are at the turning point, one is focusing resources at the point of failure and collapse. The logic of prevention suggests that resources should be focused on potentially successful situations where by putting in resources at an earlier stage, the point of collapse is not reached. Of course, the prevention argument does assume that collapse can be averted, and this is not always the case where problems primarily arise from an inexorable physiological decline as is often the case with dementia. It was not always clear whether the frequent use of the prevention argument to justify intervention before the point of collapse really arose from a belief in its logic, or whether it was mainly used as a means of buttressing a value position that found the thoroughgoing application of the turning point argument professionally and morally unacceptable.

Targeting resources exclusively on those who are on the brink will not necessarily mean targeting on the most heavily burdened or stressed. There is likely to be *some* association since subjective stress and the physical burden of caring are known to be related to an inability to continue caring, though the association is not a complete one and there are many intervening variables. Some carers who are at the point of withdrawing support may be so, less because of the burdens of caring, than from other factors such as the rival claims of other family relationships, or simply a lower level of commitment to caring. Targeting resources on those about to withdraw may involve supporting some carers who are not heavily burdened or stressed and who are at the light end of caring. It may also involve failing to support certain carers who are heavily burdened or stressed but whose commitment to the relationship is such that they will *never* withdraw their support. As a result, it is an approach that violates 'common-sense' principles of justice and equity and may as a result be politically unacceptable. This provides an additional reason why service providers do not endorse it as a practice model.

Conversely, no one operated a full *substitution system*, in the sense of providing services that would replace the input of the carer, substituting for him or her completely. This could be justified either on the basis of an extreme extension of the carer *per se* argument (freeing carers from all their burdens), or on the basis of arguments that the proper aim of services should be to enable disabled people to live free from enforced reliance on carers; as such, it embodies the model of relationship based on the superseded carer described in Chapter 2. Resources are the obvious reason for the absence of such an approach. The resource implications of a full substitution system are enormous; early attempts to shadow cost the inputs of carers have hinted at the magnitude (Nissel and Bonnerjea 1982; Wright 1987).

There are, however, additional reasons for the rejection of this approach. Certain responsibilities that carers undertake are almost impossible to provide by means of formal services, for example, getting up in the night to turn somebody who has become trapped in a particular position. The carer can occasionally be replaced by a night sitter, but unless the sitter is permanently living in the home, he or she cannot wholly substitute for the carer. As we have seen, needs that arise only periodically but in a way that require immediate response, are particularly difficult for services to meet. Were one to attempt to provide formal services to undertake these things, they would so intrude into family life as almost to negate it.

A slightly less thoroughgoing version of the substitution argument involves not attempting to substitute wholly for the carer, but treating a disabled person with a carer in exactly the same way as a disabled person without. Service allocation would thus be on a *carer-blind basis*. This would involve less input than would be the case with the full substitution version, since the disabled person living alone is unlikely to receive the level of care inputs from the formal system that they do from a carer; this is certainly the case with support in the form of company or keeping an eye on the person, but is true also of direct physical assistance. Once again no service provider operated on this basis, with the exception of certain responses to learning difficulty. This was again largely because of the resource implications. There is an almost inevitable bias in services towards targeting the unsupported. Services want to maximize welfare gains for clients. The pressure of demand means that the claims of disabled people with and without carers are competing; in judging the priority of need it is not surprising that service providers should respond to the existence of a carer.

In general service providers avoided these poles, and operated in a mixed and middle ground where instrumental approaches operated in parallel with principles that stressed the interest of the carer *per se*. Within that middle ground, service providers deployed a limited rationality, putting boundaries around the area within which they would operate according to certain professional aims and principles. This was most clearly the case with the community nurses who, as we have seen, operated an 'in-and-out' system that protected good practice by limiting its application to certain carers only. Occupational therapists operated a parallel version through their use of waiting lists; recipients were not targeted or prioritized, but those who were willing to wait eventually received the full service. This setting of boundaries enabled service providers to feel they were protecting strategic goals. This was most clearly the case with services for people with learning disabilities in Area II, where, as we have seen, the ideal of moving all adults on to independent living was the stated aim, though one that the authority lacked the resources to implement. By applying it vigorously only to certain cases it was possible to protect it as an ideal, though the discrepancy between the rhetoric and the reality provoked anger among some carers. By the same token, screening and filtering devices were of central importance in limiting demand, and thus putting a boundary around the area within which a full response would be made. Most service providers avoided case-seeking, and did not actively promote the use of their service by carers. Some, such as the home-help organizers and the community nurses, operated systems of implicit withdrawal that required carers to reassert their needs. Adopting a passive approach, as was common among GPs, again required carers to put themselves forward and make their needs known.

In addition, there were other more complex principles or models of practice structuring responses. As we have seen in the sections on the different service providers, the ways in which carers were or were not incorporated varied considerably according to the professional background and role of the practitioner, with different service providers adopting different bases for their practice in relation to carers. Some, for example, implicitly targeted their resources on an amplification model whereby they supported and educated carers in order to amplify their own input. This was most characteristic of health professionals like community nurses, but it arose also in relation to the behavioural modification programmes that attempted to recruit carers into the therapeutic regime. Others focused more openly on shortfalls, aiming to do only those things that the carer was unable to do. Fuller accounts of these various bases are contained in Chapters 4 to 6.

In Chapter 8 we concentrated not so much on how service providers constructed their practice, but how features of the caring situation affect their, and the carers', perception of appropriate intervention. Relationship, age, moral status, attitude to caring: the aims of services were clearly refracted through mediating expectations in relation to these systematic features of caring. Service providers also responded to more individually-based features of the situation. They did, for example, respond to distress in the carer where this became apparent to them (though we have noted some of the ways in which such distress might not become so). Responding to stress was widely regarded as a legitimate aim of a service, something service providers were happy to endorse as a principal guiding practice. It was not, however, pursued in any thorough-going way; also it has never achieved the legitimacy as an outcome measure that it has in some of the research literature on carers, where increasing well-being has often been used as a measure of the effectiveness of an intervention (Davies and Challis 1986; Levin *et al.* 1989; Davies *et al.* 1990).

Certain aims did receive universal approval, but these tended to be less global, more situational in character. Allowing the carer to have a holiday was the clearest example, being endorsed as a legitimate aim by all practitioners. This primarily reflected culturally-held beliefs that a break of some sort was a reasonable expectation, but it also appeared to reflect the ability of service providers to respond in this area. Allowing the carer to go on holiday occasionally was something that services could do. Services are better able to respond to one-off special needs of carers than to requirements for continual support. The problem of enabling the carer to work illustrates this, and here respondents were more equivocal. Many did endorse this as an aim, and one that extended to married women, with professionals like psychiatrists or social workers emphasizing the importance of work for well-being, and lower-status staff like home-care organizers recognizing that many women had no choice economically but to work. But some service providers gave a more qualified response, particularly where the disabled person needed constant supervision. There the general aim was compromised by the recognition that they did not have the means to enable such carers to work.

Thus there is evidence that certain outcomes, albeit of a situational rather than global nature, are widely endorsed. There is also evidence that these are in turn refracted through expectations particular to the individual: the mediating factors concerning for example, gender, age, relationship, are identified in Chapter 8. Taken together, the two can be seen as relating to a vaguely defined but embedded concept of 'normal' life. We saw this operating particularly clearly in relation to the social worker who attempted to enable Ms Myers to live what she saw as a normal life for a single woman in her thirties; or the social worker who saw Ms Arne leaving her mother's house as part of normal inter-generational conflict, part of the transition to adulthood. For some carers, however, particularly spouses, caring for a partner was itself interpreted as part of the normal expectation of marriage: bad luck that he or she needs such support, but part of what you had implicitly signed up to in marriage. These carers were not assumed to need a break from the uninterrupted company of their spouses in the way that others might. On the few occasions when service providers allow themselves to think more widely about carers' needs, it is against such ideas of 'normal life' that they do so, and what is normal is of course much dependent on who you are: your age, sex, class, relationship.

Restoring carers to what can be seen as a 'normal' expectation of life is, of course, not the overriding aim. Attempting to do so would go dangerously near the full substitution model described above that no service provider espoused. As we have noted, what was endorsed as an aim for intervention was itself affected by the practicalities of provision. Agencies endorse the kinds of outcomes that they are able to achieve, and these in turn affect how carers' needs are perceived. This brings us to the next issue within community care, that of needs-led assessment.

Needs-led assessment

A recurring theme of the recent Government guidance concerning community care has been the emphasis on needs-led assessment. One of the difficulties in considering how carers might fit into such a concept arises from the uncertainty of the meaning, or rather status, of the term. If one takes the concept of needs-led assessment seriously, as opposed to simply regarding it as a managerialist term designed to effect changes in culture but not bearing any great analytic weight, problems arise over the definition of needs. This is particularly so in the absence of any serious philosophical, cultural or politically-based discussion as to what needs are, of how they should be conceptualized, and which should legitimately be met by public welfare agencies. The term 'needs-led assessment' assumes that the nature of social welfare needs is unproblematic: that they have a clear and stable existence; that their legitimacy is unchallenged; and that the definitions of them are shared by agencies and citizens. In reality, none of these features obtains. Needs in this field are highly contentious, and in practice have always been defined in the context of a service tradition. Needs are in large measure defined by the services that exist to meet them: social welfare agencies do the kinds of things that social welfare agencies do. There is an inevitable circularity in this. The problem extends to the experiences of clients who learn through contact and the process of negotiation which needs they can legitimately express and may appropriately expect help with. We touched on this process of the social construction of need in Chapter 2, noting in particular the unequal context of power and authority in which it takes place. To this degree therefore it is artificial to attempt to disengage the definition of need wholly from the body of practice that has traditionally defined it. Needs-led assessment in the literal sense is impossible except in the context of a clearly articulated philosophy of need.

Of course the term may still have meaning. In so far as it denotes a greater flexibility, a capacity to listen to what clients say and a willingness to look more widely for solutions, it is welcome and can be meaningful. The argument, however, remains circular, though it is a large and virtuous circle rather than a small and vicious one.

How might carers fit into this? We have noted earlier how carers are a relatively new concern for social care agencies. There is not the same service tradition to draw upon in defining what needs should appropriately be recognized as there is for other client groups; the study made clear the fluid and negotiated quality of expectations in this field. As we have seen, however, in relation to targeting, certain aims did receive relatively wide endorsement; within that context, there was certainly room for more flexible responses and a more imaginative deployment of resources.

Double discretion

In Chapter 2 we emphasized the essentially discretionary nature of service delivery systems contrasting them with systems of support that rest on entitlement to benefits. Drawing on Lipsky's characterization of the street-level bureaucrat, we described how service providers, although operating within a policy and resource framework, exercise discretion in relation to individual cases. In Chapter 3 we described the difficulties that many carers and other users face in getting accurate and reliable information about the availability of various forms of support. These two features of the service system are in fact closely related, and in the discussion that follows we shall explore why this is the case.

The issue of information that has been so repeatedly identified in the research literature is not a simple one. Although much still needs to be done to provide carers and other service users with descriptions of sources of help – with A–Zs of services and leaflets in libraries and practitioners' waiting rooms – this does not resolve the central difficulty which concerns the specificity of the advice given in such material. Information sources can say *in general* what might be available in an area, but they cannot say whether it will actually be available or whether a particular carer will be eligible to receive it. The reason for this lies in the discretionary nature of service allocation. In this area, users and carers face what we term 'double discretion'. The first form of discretion is the familiar one: service providers make discretionary judgments about individual cases. The process is all the more complex and discretionary in relation to carers in that service providers are having to make judgments about stress, volition, motivation – about 'subjective' aspects of the situation. As we noted in Chapter 2, these do not have the same 'objective' quality as do questions of mobility or visual impairment. It is hard to turn them into clear criteria of eligibility; they are by their nature open to alteration in the light of the situation. The position with carers is further complicated by the fact that *two* people's interests are involved, and these can be in conflict. These features reinforce the significance of discretion in relation to carers.

The second level of discretion relates to the fact that allocations are made in the context of specific resources. If we take the example of the community nursing service, decisions about the availability of support with, for example a bath, were clearly made in the context of individual case loads. This adds a second element of discretion to that concerning the initial assessment of the situation. Judgments are particular not just to the case but to the circumstances of the service provider: on another occasion the decision might be different. This makes it almost impossible to provide carers with definitive information as to what help is available locally and whether they are eligible to receive it. It also underlies the inability of service providers to accept the assessments of other service providers: one of the main stumbling blocks in integrating services across sectoral boundaries.

These characteristics of allocation are reinforced in the case of carers by the fact that they are helped to a large extent 'on the margins'. The marginal nature of much service response arises partly from the secondary relation that we analysed in Chapter 2 whereby carers are rarely the straightforward focus of an intervention, and partly from the incremental and marginal way in which developments occur within organizations. Carers have arrived late on the scene in the politics of service delivery; in so far as their needs have been met, it has tended to be through the deployment of marginal resources. Respite, for example, is often created out of spare resources in a residential home or hospital ward. Carer support groups often draw on the marginal resources, and good will, of individual practitioners.

Carers, of course, gain from this use of resources, in the sense that they do receive *some* support. Service providers can rightly see this in a positive light: they are meeting the needs of at least some carers, and it is better that this should happen than that no carers should be helped. This sentiment ran through the comments of a number of service providers. It underpinned the reaction of a home-help organizer who when asked about priorities responded that her staff 'worked very hard' and 'did what they could'. It underlay the distinctive use of the term 'flexible' by home-help organizers and community nurse managers that we noted earlier.

This pattern of marginal use can produce problems for carers. Sometimes the service provided was not well geared to their needs. This can be the case in relation to short-term care, where the creation of respite out of marginal hospital or residential care resources produces a service ill-adapted to the needs of users. Carers also experienced problems over uncertainty of provision. For example, as we have seen, the community nursing service gives priority to acute medical interventions, with the result that the provision of baths is left to the end of the shift, where it is often completely displaced by the other work. As a result the service cannot guarantee the provision of a bath, to the frustration of the carer. From the nursing management viewpoint, this pattern of work represents the most effective use of the marginal time of a trained nurse. Using marginal resources maximizes deployment and is, in some cases, the only way that carers receive support. However, it disrupts the imposition of a stable or 'rational' system of allocation and makes impossible attempts to provide clear information about availability. This leads us to our final theme, that of transparency.

Transparency

One of the expressed aims of the new community care has been that of greater transparency. Transparency involves making explicit the detailed aims and priorities of the organization so that the reasons why decisions are made and the bases for judgments become open – transparent to view. Within Conservative thinking, it has been exemplified by the *Citizen's Charter* and related customer charters for public services. Such approaches deploy the language of consumerism, asserting the right to fuller information in order to pursue choices and enforce a reasonable level of service. The Left has also expressed a concern for greater transparency, although articulated within a different framework, one emphasizing entitlement, the rights of citizenship and the importance of user views.

Few would quarrel with such a principle: it makes the system open, and thus open to challenge; it requires consistency, and with that equity of response; it clarifies objectives and encourages the strategic pursuit of them. Problems come, however, from the fact that the service welfare system has historically never been run on this basis. It was clear from our analysis, for example, that service providers were not imposing consistent systems of targeting. This was not simply because of the complexities of human situations that disrupt what Lipsky terms the 'application of programmatic formats', or the vagaries of service providers who 'fail' to maintain consistency between cases. It was because service providers did not want to apply a wholly consistent approach. Resources for carers are very short. As we have seen, were service providers to determine clear target groups that would define which carers should receive priority, the numbers covered would be very small. Indeed, we can surmise that only those who were 'on the brink' *and* very heavily stressed would receive any support. Carrying through a fully-rationalized model of allocation and response would threaten the values held by professionals.

Such a clarification of targets raises serious political problems. The service system has always relied on the fragmentation of decisions in ways that have obscured its aims. As with health care, the tradition has always been one of cutting up the corpse so fine that it cannot be seen. Being explicit as to aims and as to who does and does not get help is potentially destabilizing. Systematic randomness of response blurs the pattern in ways that allow the system to survive. Indeterminacy of aims arises not simply from the failure of managers to set targets but also from factors functional to the organization. Welfare services have a number of functions – symbolic functions, masking functions – that are not about achieving states of welfare. It remains open to question therefore how far it is possible to make the criteria of response fully transparent and rationalized without exposing the system to a degree of conflict that would undermine its legitimacy.

Conclusion

Carers have come late to the politics of service delivery. As a result, any thorough shake-up of the old system offers considerable opportunities for them and for the incorporation of their needs and interests into service delivery. The carer issue has been an increasingly prominant one. The documentation relating to the new community care refers to carers extensively, and it is increasingly common for policy documents at local as well as national level to describe their needs as part of the legitimate concerns of service provision. How far the new community care will in fact embody a radically different approach to service delivery is still unclear. Much remains to be clarified, particularly in relation to the levels and patterns of funding. Changes in other sectors, notably the acute medical sector, though also in the structure of local government, may force the pace of change, but they may also, ironically, inhibit real change. Where carers will fit into this is similarly unclear. What remains certain, however, is that they will continue to provide the majority of care, and that how they are perceived by service providers will continue to determine the level and pattern of help they will receive in doing so.

APPENDIX

The book draws on an empirical study funded by the Department of Health and undertaken at the Social Policy Research Unit, University of York. The two research reports published by SPRU contain an account of the methodology of the study (Twigg and Atkin, with Perring 1990b; Twigg and Atkin 1991). They also contain a much fuller account of the analysis, of the individual cases and patterns of response. The conclusions presented in this book draw on that more detailed base.

Obtaining the sample of carers

The sample of carers was obtained by drawing on earlier, large-scale studies of disabled people that had been undertaken in the two study areas. These offered the considerable advantage of representing natural populations rather than ones generated through the records of service providers. Many studies of carers have been forced to rely on the service provider route, and this has compromised the ability to generalize their findings. Many carers are not in touch with services and, as we have seen, service providers are often unaware of their existence.

The carer sample

A total of 90 carers were interviewed and, divided equally between the two areas, Areas I and II, classified according to the client or patient group of the cared-for person. The study was confined to carers who shared a household with the cared-for person. The numbers were as follows:

Carers of:	
adults with a learning disability	18
adults with mental health problems	20
adults with physical disabilities	16
older people with physical disabilities	20
older people with mental infirmity	16
Total	90

Obtaining the service provider sample

The sample of service providers was generated by asking individual carers to identify their most significant service contacts. In some cases this generated more than one interview; in a small number of cases, none. We thus tracked from the carer to the service provider and did not pre-empt which service providers were important to carers.

The service provider sample

A total of 125 interviews were undertaken with service providers and managers. The service providers covered 46 health authority staff, 48 local authority staff and 12 non-statutory staff. The research team also spoke to 35 service managers: 16 in health authorities; 13 in local authorities; 6 in the voluntary sector.

The interviews

Both the carer and service practitioner interviews were qualitative in character, and conducted by cueing and prompting the respondent towards a detailed exposition of the situation. The interviews were recorded and transcribed. The researchers conducted all the interviews themselves.

The two areas

The study was undertaken in two areas, designated Area I and Area II, in the north of England. It was not based on an experimental design and the two areas were chosen simply to reflect variation. The areas had similar demographic and material environments. Both were areas of declining heavy industry with higher than national average unemployment figures. Their demographic profiles were similar.

REFERENCES

Abrams, P., Abrams, S., Humphrey, R. and Snaith, R. (1989) *Neighbourhood Care and Social Policy*, London, HMSO.

Allen, I.C. (1983) *Short-Stay Residential Care for the Elderly*, London, Policy Studies Institute.

Anderson, D., Lait, J. and Marsland, D. (1981) *Breaking the Spell of the Welfare State: Strategies for Reducing Public Expenditure*, London, Social Affairs Unit.

Anderson, D. and Dawson, G. (eds) (1986) *Family Portraits*, London, Social Affairs Unit.

Anderson, M. (1971) *Family Structure in Nineteenth Century Lancashire*, Cambridge, Cambridge University Press.

Anderson, M. (1980) *Approaches to the History of the Western Family: 1500–1914*, London, Macmillan.

Arber, S. and Ginn, J. (1991) *Gender and Later Life: A Sociological Analysis of Resources and Constraints*, London, Sage.

Arber, S., Gilbert, N. and Evandrou, M. (1988) Gender, household composition and receipt of domiciliary services by the elderly disabled, *Journal of Social Policy*, 17(2).

Atkin, K. (1991) Health, illness, disability and black minorities: a speculative critique of present day discourse, *Disability, Handicap and Society*, 6(1).

Atkin, K. and Rollings, J. (1993) *Community Care in a Multi-Racial Britain: A Critical Review of the Literature*, London, HMSO.

Atkinson, F.I. and McHaffie, H.E. (1992a) *A Systematic Approach to Assessing Carers' Needs and Providing Nursing Support: An Evaluation of Outcomes*, Edinburgh, Nursing Research Unit, University of Edinburgh.

Atkinson, F.I. and McHaffie, H.E. (1992b) Addressing the needs of informal carers: a neglected area of nursing practice, *Journal of Advanced Nursing*, 14.

Audit Commission (1986) *Making a Reality of Community Care*, London, HMSO.

Audit Commission (1989) *Developing Community Care for Adults with a Mental Handicap*, Occasional Paper No. 9, London, Audit Commission for Local Authorities in England and Wales.

Badger, F., Cameron, E. and Evers, H. (1989) The nursing auxiliary service and care of elderly patients, *Journal of Advanced Nursing*, 14.

Baldwin, S.M. (1985) *The Costs of Caring: Families with Disabled Children*, London, Routledge and Kegan Paul.

Baldwin, S. and Twigg, J. (1991) Women and community care: reflections on a debate, in *Women's Issues in Social Policy*, edited by Maclean, M. and Groves, D., London, Routledge.

Bank-Mikkelson, N.E. (1969) *Changing Patterns in Residential Services for the Mentally Retarded*, Washington DC, President's Committee on Mental Retardation.

Barclay Committee (1982) *Social Workers: Their Role and Tasks*, London, NISW.

Barrett, S. and Fudge, C. (1981) *Policy and Action: Essays on the Implementation of Public Policy*, London, Methuen.

Barrowclough, C. and Tarrier, N. (1984) Psychosocial interventions with families and their effects on the course of schizophrenia: a review, *Psychological Medicine*, 14.

Bateson, G., Jackson, D., Haley, J. and Weakland, J. (1956) Towards a theory of schizophrenia, *Behavioural Sciences*, 1.

Bayley, M. (1973) *Mental Handicap and Community Care*, London, Routledge and Kegan Paul.

Bayley, M. (1982) Helping care to happen in the city, in *Community Care: The Family, the State and Social Policy*, edited by Walker, A., Oxford, Blackwell.

Bebbington, A.C. and Kelly, A. (1992) *Trends in Unit Costs for Local Authority Personal Social Services*, Kent, University of Kent, PSSRU.

Bebbington, A.C., Charnley, H., Davies, B.P. *et al.* (1986) *The Domiciliary Care Project: Meeting the Needs of the Elderly*, Interim Report, Kent, University of Kent, PSSRU.

Blannin, J. (1987) Incontinence: men's problems, *Community Outlook*, February.

Blaxter, M. (1976) *The Meaning of Disability*, London, Heinemann.

Blaxter, M. and Pearson, E. (1982) *Mothers and Daughters: A Three Generational Study of Health Attitudes and Behaviour*, London, Heinemann.

Blom-Cooper, L. (1989) *Occupational Therapy: An Emerging Profession in Health Care*, London, Duckworth.

Bourne, S. and Lewis, E. (1977) Doctors despair: a paradox of progress, *Journal of the Royal College of General Practitioners*, 27.

Bradshaw, J. (1980) *The Family Fund: An Initiative in Social Policy*, London, Routledge and Kegan Paul.

Brearley, P. and Mandelstram, M. (1992) *A Review of Literature 1986–1991 on Day Care Services for Adults*, London, HMSO.

Briggs, A. and Oliver, J. (1985) *Caring: Experiences of Looking after Disabled Relatives*, London, Routledge and Kegan Paul.

Brocklehurst, J.C. and Tucker, J.S. (1980) *Progress in Geriatric Day Care*, London, The King's Fund.

Brody, E.M. (1981) Women in the middle and family help to older people, *Gerontologist*, 21(5).

Brook, P. and Jestice, S. (1986) Relief for the demented and their relatives, *Geriatric Medicine*, June.

Brooker, C. (1990) All in the family?, *Nursing Times*, 86(2).

Brown, G.W., Birley, J.L.T. and Wing, J.K. (1972) The influence of family life on the course of schizophrenic disorders: a replication, *British Journal of Psychiatry*, 13.

Brown, G.W. and Harris, T.O. (1978) *Social Origins of Depression: A Study of Psychiatric Disorder in Women*, London, Tavistock Publications.

Buckquet, D. and Curtis, S. (1986) Socio-demographic variation in perceived illness and the use of primary care, *Social Science and Medicine*, 23.

Bulmer, M. (1986) *Neighbours: the Work of Philip Abrams*, Cambridge, Cambridge University Press.

Byrne, E.A. and Cunningham, C.C. (1985) The effects of mentally handicapped children on families, *Journal of Child Psychology and Psychiatry*, 26(6).

Byrne, P.S. and Long, B.E. (1976) *Doctors Talking to Patients*, London, HMSO.

Carr, J. (1976) Effect on the family of a child with Down's syndrome, *Physiotherapy*, 62(1).

Carter, J. (1981) *Day Services for Adults: Somewhere to Go*, London, Allen and Unwin.

Challis, D. and Davies, B. (1986) *Case Management in Community Care*, Aldershot, Gower.

Challis, D. and Ferlie, E. (1986) Changing patterns of fieldwork organisation: the headquarter's view, *British Journal of Social Work*, 16.

Challis, D. and Ferlie, E. (1987) Changing patterns of fieldwork organisation: the team leaders' view, *British Journal of Social Work*, 17.

Challis, D. and Ferlie, E. (1988) The myth of general practice: specialisation in social work, *Journal of Social Policy*, 17.

Connolly, N. (1988) *Caring in the Multi-racial Community*, London, Policy Studies Institute.

Creer, C. (1975) Living with schizophrenia, *Social Work Today*, 6.

Creer, C. and Wing, J.K. (1974) *Schizophrenia at Home*, Surbiton, National Schizophrenia Fellowship.

Creer, C., Sturt, E. and Wykes, T. (1982) The role of relatives, in 'Long-term community care experience in a London borough', *Psychological Medicine*, 12, monograph supplement 2, edited by Wing, J.K.

Crombie, D.L. (1984) *Social Class and Health Status: Inequality of Difference*, Occasional Paper 25, London, The Royal College of General Practitioners.

Dalley, G. (1988) *Ideologies of Caring: Rethinking Community and Collectivism*, London, Macmillan.

Dant, T. and Gearing, B. (1990) Keyworkers for elderly people in the community: case managers and care co-ordinators, *Journal of Social Policy*, 19.

Davies, B. and Bebbington, A.C. (1983) Equity and efficiency in the allocation of personal social services, *Journal of Social Policy*, 12(3).

Davies, B. and Challis, D. (1986) *Matching Resources to Needs in Community Care*, Aldershot, Gower.

Davies, B., Bebbington, A., Charnley, H. *et al.* (1990) *Resources, Needs and Outcomes in Community Based Care*, Aldershot, Avebury.

Davis, A. (1984) Day care, in *Social Work in Mental Health*, edited by Olsen, M.R., London, Tavistock.

Delphy, C. and Leonard, D. (1992) *Familiar Exploitation: A New Analysis of Marriage in Comtemporary Western Societies*, Cambridge, Polity Press.

Department of Health (1990) *Community Care in the Next Decade and Beyond: Policy Guidance*, London, HMSO.

Department of Health and Social Security (1980) *Mental Handicap: Progress, Problems and Priorities*, London, HMSO.

Dexter, M. and Herbert, W. (1983) *The Home Help Service*, London, Tavistock.

Dingwall, R. (1977) *Social Organization of Health Visitor Training*, London, Croom Helm.

Dingwall, R., Raffety, A.M. and Webster, C. (1988) *An Introduction to the Social History of Nursing*, London, Routledge.

Dunnell, K. and Dobbs, J. (1982) *Nurses Working in the Community*, London, OPCS.

Ellard, J. (1974) The disease of being a doctor, *Medical Journal of Australia*, ii.

Elmore, R. (1981) Backwards mapping: implementation research and policy decisions, *Political Science Quarterly*, 94(4).

Equal Opportunities Commission (1980) *The Experience of Caring for Elderly and Handicapped Dependants: Survey Report*, Manchester, EOC.

Evandrou, M., Arber, S., Dale, A. and Gilbert, G.N. (1986) Who cares for the elderly: family care provision and receipt of statutory services, in *Dependency and Interdependency in Old Age*, edited by Phillipson, C., Bernard, M. and Strang, P., London, Croom Helm.

Fadden, G., Bebbington, P. and Kuipers, L. (1987) Caring and its burdens: a study of relatives of depressed patients, *British Journal of Psychiatry*, 150.

Falloon, I.R.H., Boyd, J.L., McGill, G.W. *et al.* (1982) Family management in the prevention of exacerbations of schizophrenia: a controlled study, *New England Journal of Medicine*, 306.

Fennell, G., Emerson, A.R., Sidell, M. and Hague, A. (1981) *Day Centres for the Elderly in East Anglia*, Norwich, Centre for East Anglian Studies.

Finch, J. (1989) *Family Obligations and Social Change*, Cambridge, Polity Press.

Finch, J. and Groves, D. (1980) Community care and the family: a case for equal opportunities, *Journal of Social Policy*, 9(4).

Finch, J. and Groves, D. (1983) *A Labour of Love: Women, Work and Caring*, London, Routledge and Kegan Paul.

Finch, J. and Mason, J. (1993) *Negotiating Family Responsibilities*, London, Routledge.

Flynn, N. (1989) The New Right and social policy, *Policy and Politics*, 17(2).

Friedson, E. (1970) *Profession of Medicine: A Study of the Sociology of Applied Knowledge*, New York, Mead and Co.

Froland, C. (1981) Formal and informal care: discontinuities in a continuum, *Social Service Review*, S4.

Gibbons, J.S., Horn, S.M., Powell, J.M. and Gibbons, J.L. (1984) Schizophrenic patients and their families: a survey in a psychiatric service based on a DGH unit, *British Journal of Psychiatry*, 144.

Gilhooly, M. (1982) Social aspects of senile dementia, in *Current Trends in Gerontology: Proceedings of the 1980 Conference of the British Society of Gerontology*, edited by Taylor, R. and Gilmore, A., Aldershot, Gower.

Gilleard, C.J., Gilleard, E., Gledhill, K. and Whittick, J. (1984) Caring for the elderly mentally infirm at home: a survey of the supporters, *Journal of Epidemiology and Community Health*, 38.

Gilligan, C. (1982) *In a Different Voice: Psychological Theory and Women's Development*, Cambridge, MA, Harvard University Press.

Glendinning, C. (1983) *Unshared Care*, London, Routledge and Kegan Paul.

Glendinning, C. (1985) *A Single Door*, London, George Allen and Unwin.

Glendinning, C. (1992) *The Costs of Informal Care: Looking Inside the Household*, London, HMSO. employment

Glennerster, H. and Matsaganis, M. (1991) *A Foothold for Fundholding: A Preliminary Report on the Introduction of GP Fundholding*, London, Suntory Toyota International Centre for Economics and Related Disciplines, London School of Economics.

Glew, J. (1986) Continence a woman's lot?, *Nursing Times*, 9 April.

Glosser, G. and Wexler, D. (1985) Participants evaluation of educational/support groups for families of patients with Alzheimer's disease and other dementias, *Gerontologist*, 25(3).

Goldberg, E.M. and Warburton, R.W. (1979) *Ends and Means in Social Work*, London, Allen and Unwin.

Goldman, H. (1980) The post hospital mental patient and family therapy, *The Journal of Marital and Family Therapy*, 6.

Goodwin, S. (1988) Whither health visiting?, *Health Visitor*, 61(12).

Grad, J. and Sainsbury, P. (1963) Mental illness and the family, *Lancet*, i.

Graham, H. (1983) Caring: labour of love, in *A Labour of Love: Women, Work and Caring*, edited by Finch, J. and Groves, D., London, Routledge and Kegan Paul.

Graham, H. (1991) The concept of caring in feminist research: the case of domestic service, *Sociology*, 25(1).

Graham, J. (1984) *Take Up of FIS: Knowledge, Attitudes and Experience – Claimants and Non-Claimants*, Stormont, PPRU.

Green, H. (1988) *General Household Survey 1985: Informal Carers*, London, HMSO.

Gubrium, J.F. (1989) Local cultures and service policy, in *The Politics of Field Research: Sociology Beyond Enlightenment*, edited by Gubrium, J.F. and Silverman, D., London, Sage.

Ham, C. and Hill, M. (1984) *The Policy Process in the Modern Capitalist State*, Brighton, Wheatsheaf.

Harris, C. (1987) The individual and society: a processial approach, in *Rethinking the Life Cycle*, edited by Brymar, A., Bytheway, B., Allat, P. and Keil, T., London, Macmillan.

Hasselkus, B.R. and Brown, M. (1983) *The Forgotten Army: Family Care and Elderly People*, London, Family Policy Studies Centre.

Herzlich, C. (1973) *Health and Illness: A Social Psychological Analysis*, London, Academic Press.

Hettiaratchy, P. and Manthorpe, J. (1992) Group physiotherapy supporting the carers of elderly mentally ill people, in *Care Giving in Dementia: Research and Applications*, edited by Jones, G. and Miesen, G.M.L., London, Wiley.

Hills, D. (1991) *Carer Support in the Community: Evaluation of the Department of Health Initiative; Demonstration Districts for Informal Carers 1986–1989*, London, HMSO.

Hinrichsen, G.A., Revenson, T.A. and Shinn, M. (1985) Does self-help help? An empirical investigation of scoliosis peer support group, *Journal of Social Issues*, 41(1).

Hirst, M. (1984) *Moving On: Transfer from Child to Adult services for Young People with Disabilities*, Social Policy Research Unit, DSS 190, University of York.

Hirst, M.A. (1990) Financial independence and social security, *Children and Society*, 4(1).

Hochschild, A. (1983) *The Managed Heart: The Commercialization of Human Feelings*, Berkley, CA, University of California.

Holland, B. and Lewando-Hundt, G. (1987) *Coventry Ethnic Minorities Elderly Survey: Method, Data and Applied Action*, Coventry, City of Coventry Ethnic Development Unit.

Hooyman, N.R. (1990) Women as caregivers of the elderly: implications for social welfare policy and practice, in *Aging and Caregiving: Theory, Research and Policy*, edited by Biegel, D.E. and Blum, A., London, Sage.

Hubert, J. (1990) At home and alone: families and young adults with challenging behaviour, in *Better Lives: Changing Services for People with Learning Difficulties*, edited by Booth, T., Sheffield, Joint Unit for Social Services Research/Community Care.

Hunter, D.J., McKeganey, N.P. and MacPherson, I.A. (1988) *Care of the Elderly: Policy and Practice*, Aberdeen, Aberdeen University Press.

Huntingdon, J. (1981) *Social Work and General Medical Practice*, London, Allen and Unwin.

Hyman, M. (1977) *The Extra Costs of Disabled Living*, London, DIG/ARC.

Jaehnig, W. (1979) A family service for the mentally handicapped, *Fabian Society Tract*, No. 460, London, Fabian Society.

James, N. (1989) Emotional labour: skill and work in the social regulation of feelings, *Sociological Review*, 37(1).

Johnson, M. and Cross, M. (1983) Race and primary health care in the West Midlands, *Radical Community Medicine*, 16.

Johnstone, E.C., Owens, D.G.C., Gold, A. *et al.* (1984) Schizophrenic patients discharged from hospital – a follow-up study, *British Journal of Psychiatry*, 145.

Jones, D.A. and Vetter, N.J. (1984) A survey of those who care for the elderly at home: their problems and their needs, *Social Science and Medicine*, 19(5).

Jones, N. (1988) *A Report to the Department on the Attitudes of Older Carers of Mentally Handicapped Adults Living in the Borough*, Hammersmith and Fulham Social Service Department.

Joshi, H. (1987) The cost of caring, in *Women and Poverty*, edited by Glendinning, C. and Millar, J., Brighton, Wheatsheaf.

Kelson, N. (1985) *The Short-Term Care Project, Eastern Countries: Final Report to the Welfare Advisory Panel*, London, Parkinson's Disease Society.

Kerr, S. (1982) Deciding about supplementary pensions: a provisional model, *Journal of Social Policy*, 11.

Kiple, K.F. and King, V.I.H. (1981) *Another Dimension to the Black Diaspora*, Cambridge, Cambridge University Press.

Knapp, M. (1984) *The Economics of Social Care*, London, Macmillan.

Kreisman, D. and Joy, V. (1974) Family response to the mental illness of a relative: a review of the literature, *Schizophrenia Bulletin*, 10(7a 11).

Kuipers, L. (1979) Expressed emotion: a review, *British Journal of Social and Clinical Psychology*, 18.

Laing, R.D. (1960) *The Divided Self: An Existential Study in Sanity and Madness*, Harmondsworth, Penguin.

Laing, W. (1991) *Empowering the Elderly: Direct Consumer Funding of Care Services*, London, IEA Health and Welfare Unit.

Land, H. (1978) Who cares for the family, *Journal of Social Policy*, 7(3).

Land, H. and Rose, H. (1985) Compulsory altruism for some or an altruistic society for all, in *In Defence of Welfare*, edited by Bean, P., Ferris, J. and Whynes, D., London, Tavistock.

Laslett, T.P.R. (ed.) (1972) *Household and Family in Past Time*, Cambridge, Cambridge University Press.

Laslett, T.P.R. (1977) *Family Life and Illicit Love in Earlier Generations*, Cambridge, Cambridge University Press.

Leat, D. (1990) *For Love and Money: The Role of Payment in Encouraging the Provision of Care*, York, Joseph Rowntree Foundation.

Leat, D. (1992) Innovations and special schemes, in *Carers: Research and Practice*, edited by Twigg, J., London, HMSO.

Levin, E., Sinclair, I. and Gorbach, P. (1989) *Families, Services and Confusion in Old Age*, Aldershot, Gower.

Lewis, J. and Meredith, B. (1988) *Daughters Who Care: Daughters Caring for Mothers at Home*, London, Routledge and Kegan Paul.

Lidz, T. (1968) The family language and the transmission of schizophrenia, in *The Transmission of Schizophrenia*, edited by Rosenthal, T. and Kety, S., Oxford, Pergamon.

Lipsky, M. (1980) *Street Level Bureaucracy*, New York, Russell Sage.

Litwak, E. and Kulis, S. (1983) Changes in helping networks with changes in the health of old people: social policy and social theory, in *Evaluating the Welfare State*, edited by Spiro, S. and Yuchtman-Yaer E., New York, Academic Press.

Lovelock, R. (1985) *Against the Tide: Approaches to the Domiciliary Support of Frail Elderly People in Hampshire*, Portsmouth, SSRIU.

Luker, K.A. (1979) Health visiting and the elderly, *Midwife, Health Visitor and Community Nurse*, 15(11).

Mackintosh, S., Mearns, R. and Leather, P. (1990) *Housing in Later Life: The Housing Finance Implications of an Ageing Society*, University of Bristol, School of Advanced Urban Studies.

Mandelstrom, D. (ed.) (1981) *Incontinence and its Management*, London, Croom Helm.

Martin, J. and Wright, A. (1988) *The Financial Circumstances of Disabled Adults Living in Private Households*, London, HMSO.

Mayer, J.E. and Timms, N. (1970) *The Client Speaks: Working Class Impressions of Casework*, London, Routledge and Kegan Paul.

McGrath, M. (1991) *Multi-disciplinary Teamwork: Community Mental Handicap Teams*, Aldershot, Avebury.

McGrath, M. and Grant, G. (1992) Supporting 'needs-led' services: implications for planning and management services, *Journal of Social Policy*, 21(1).

McLachlan, S., Sheard, D. and Anderson, K. (1985) Relatives' open evenings can help, *Health and Social Services Journal*, 15 November.

McLaughlin, E. (1991) *Social Security and Community Care: The Case of the Invalid Care Allowance: Final Report*, DSS Research Report Series No. 4, London, HMSO.

Mechanic, D. (1970) Correlates of frustration among British general practitioners, *Journal of Social Behaviour*, 11(2).

Moroney, R.M. (1976) *The Family and the State: Considerations for Social Policy*, London, Longman.

Morris, J. (1991) *Pride Against Prejudice: Transforming Attitudes to Disability*, London, Women's Press.

Nirje, B. (1970) The normalisation principle – implications and comments, *British Journal of Mental Subnormality*, 16.

Nissel, M. and Bonnerjea, L. (1982) *Family Care of the Handicapped Elderly: Who Pays?*, London, Policy Studies Institute.

Nolan, M.R. and Grant, G. (1989) Addressing the needs of informal carers: a neglected area of nursing practice, *Journal of Advanced Nursing*, 14.

Norman, A. (1985) *Triple Jeopardy: Growing Old in a Second Homeland*, Policy Studies in Ageing No. 3, London, Centre for Policy on Ageing.

Norton, C. (1986) Continence promoting research, *Nursing Times*, 9 April.

Oldman, C. (1990) *Moving in Old Age: New Directions in Housing Policy*, London, HMSO.

Oldman, C. (1991) *Paying for Care: Personal Sources of Funding Care*, York, Joseph Rowntree Foundation.

Oliver, M. (1990) *The Politics of Disablement*, London, Macmillan.

Olsen, M. and Rolf, W. (1984) Social perspectives of mental disorder, in *Social Work and Mental Health*, edited by Olsen, M. and Rolf, W., London, Tavistock.

Oswin, M. (1984) *They Keep Going Away: A Critical Study of Short-Term Residential Care Services for Children Who are Mentally Handicapped*, King Edward's Hospital Fund for London.

Parker, G. (1990a) *With Due Care and Attention: A Review of Research on Informal Care*, 2nd edn, London, Family Policy Studies Centre.

Parker, G. (1990b) Whose care? Whose costs? Whose benefit? A critical review of research in case management, *Ageing and Society*, 10.

Parker, G. (1992) Counting care: numbers and types of informal carers in *Carers, Research and Practice*, edited by Twigg, J., London, HMSO.

Parker, G. (1993) *With This Body: Caring and Disability in Marriage*, Buckingham, Open University Press.

Parker, G. and Lawton, D. (1990a) *Further Analysis of the 1985* General Household Survey *Data on Informal Care. Report 1: A Typology of Caring*, Social Policy Research Unit, Working Paper DHSS 715, 12.90, University of York.

Parker, G. and Lawton, D. (1990b) *Further Analysis of the 1985* General Household Survey *Data on Informal Care. Report 2: The Consequences of Caring*, Social Policy Research Unit, Working Paper DHSS 716, 12.90, University of York.

Parker, R. (1981) Tending and social policy, in *A New Look at the Personal Social Services*, edited by Goldberg, E.M. and Hatch, S., London, Policy Studies Institute.

Perring, C., Atkin, K. and Twigg, J. (1990) *Families Caring for People Diagnosed as Mentally Ill: The Literature Re-Examined*, London, HMSO.

Quine, L. and Pahl, J. (1985) Examining the causes of stress in families with severely mentally handicapped children, *British Journal of Social Work*, 15.

Quine, L. and Pahl, J. (1989) *Stress and Coping in Families Caring for a Child with Severe Mental Handicap: A Longitudinal Study*, Canterbury, Institute of Social and Applied Psychology and Centre for Health Services Studies, University of Kent.

Qureshi, H. and Walker, A. (1989) *The Caring Relationship: Elderly People and Their Families*, Basingstoke, Macmillan.

Race, D. (1987) Normalisation: theory and practice, in *Reassessing Community Care*, edited by Malin, N., London, Croom Helm.

Rai, G.S., Biclawska, C., Murphy, P.J. and Wright, G. (1986) Hazards for elderly people admitted to respite and social care, *British Medical Journal*, 292(6515).

Ramdas, A. (1986) Getting it Right: Women Carers of the Frail Elderly: An Analysis of Experiences and Support Service Needs, MA Thesis, University of York.

Richardson, A. and Higgins, R. (1992) *The Limits of Case Management: Lessons from the Wakefield Case Management Project*, Leeds, Nuffield Institute.

Richman, J. (1987) *Medicine and Health*, London, Longman.

Ritchie, J. and Mathews, A. (1982) *Take up of Rent Allowances: An In-Depth Study*, London, Social and Community Planning Research.

Robinson, J. (1985) Health visiting and health, in *Political Issues in Nursing: Past, Present and Future*, edited by White, R., Chichester, John Wiley.

Robinson, R. (1978) *In Worlds Apart: Professionals and Their Clients in the Welfare State*, London, Bedford Square Press.

Robinson, B. and Thurner, M. (1979) Taking care of aged parents: a family cycle transition, *Gerontologist*, 19.

Robinson, C. and Stalker, K. (1992) *New Directions: Suggestions for Interesting Service Development in Respite Care*, London, The King's Fund Centre.

Rojek, C., Peacock, G. and Collins, S. (1988) *Social Work and Received Ideas*, London, Routledge.

Rooney, B. (1987) *Racism and Resistance to Change: A Study of the Black Social Workers Project in Liverpool SSD*, Liverpool, University of Liverpool Sociology Department.

Rowlings, C. (1981) *Social Work with Elderly People*, London, Allen and Unwin.

Sarri, R.C. and Hasenfeld, Y. (1978) *Management of Human Services*, New York, Columbia University Press.

Scrivens, E. (1983) Rationing resources: the work of local authority occupational therapists, *British Journal of Occupational Therapy*, 46(1).

Sinclair, I. (1990) Carers: their contribution and quality of life, in *The Kaleidoscope of Care: A Review of Research of Welfare Provision for Elderly People*, edited by Sinclair, I., Parker, R., Leat, D. and Williams, J., London, HMSO.

Sinclair, I., Parker, R., Leat, D. and Williams, J. (1990) *The Kaleidoscope of Care: A Review of Welfare Provision for Elderly People*, London, HMSO.

Smith, G. and Cantley, C. (1985) *Assessing Health Care: A Study in Organisational Evaluation*, Milton Keynes, Open University Press.

Smith, G. and May, D. (1980) The artificial debate between rationalist and incrementalist models of decision making, *Policy and Politics*, 8(2).

Smith, R.M. (1984) The structured dependence of the elderly as a recent development: some sceptical historical thoughts, *Ageing and Society*, 4(4).

Smyth, M. and Robus, N. (1989) *The Financial Circumstances of Families with Disabled Children Living in Private Households*, London, HMSO.

Social Services Inspectorate (1987a) *Care for a Change? Inspection of Short-Term Care in the Personal Social Services*, London, Social Services Inspectorate, Department of Health and Social Security.

Social Services Inspectorate (1987b) *From Home Help to Home Care: An Analysis of Policy, Resourcing and Service Management*, London, Social Services Inspectorate, Department of Health and Social Security.

Social Services Inspectorate (1988) *Managing Policy Change in Home Help Services*, London, Social Services Inspectorate, Department of Health and Social Security.

Sontag, S. (1983) *Illness as Metaphor*, Harmondsworth, Penguin.

Stephens, S.A. and Christiansen, J.B. (1986) *Informal Care of the Elderly*, Lexington, MA, Lexington Books.

Stewart, J. (1986) *The New Management of Local Government*, London, Allen and Unwin.

Stimson, G.V. and Webb, B. (1975) *Going to See the Doctor: The Consultation Process in General Practice*, London, Routledge and Kegan Paul.

Thompson, E.H. and Doll, W. (1982) The burden of families coping with the mentally ill: an invisible crisis, *Family Relations: Journal of Applied Family and Child Studies*, 35(3).

Thomson, D. (1991) The welfare of the elderly in the past: a family or a community responsibility? in *Life, Death and the Elderly: Historical Perspectives*, edited by Pelling, M. and Smith, R.M., London, Routledge.

Thornton, P. (1989) *Creating a Break: A Home Care Relief Scheme for Elderly People and Their Supporters*, Mitcham, Age Concern England.

Thornton, P. (1991) Subject to contract? Volunteers as providers of community care for elderly people and their supporters, *Journal of Ageing Studies*, 5(2).

Thornton, P. and Moore, J. (1980) *The Placement of Elderly People in Private Households: An Analysis of Current Provision*, University of Leeds, Department of Social Policy and Administration Monograph.

Toseland, R.W., Labrecque, M.S., Goebel, S.T. and Whitney, M.H. (1992) An evaluation of a group program for spouses of frail elderly veterans, *Gerontologist*, xx, x.

Twigg, J. (1989a) Models of carers: how do social care agencies conceptualise their relationship with informal carers, *Journal of Social Policy*, 18(1).

Twigg, J. (1989b) Not taking the strain, *Community Care*, 27 July.

Twigg, J. (1990a) Carers of elderly people: models for analysis, in *Contrasting European Policies for the Care of Older People*, edited by Jamieson, A. and Illsley, R., Aldershot, Gower.

Twigg, J. (1990b) Personal care and the interface between the district nursing and home help services, in *Needs, Resources and Outcomes*, edited by Davies, B.P., Bebbington, A.C. and Charnley, H., Gower, Aldershot.

Twigg, J. (ed.) (1992) *Carers: Research and Practice*, London, HMSO.

Twigg, J. (1993) Integrating carers into the service system: six strategic responses, *Ageing and Society*, 13(2).

Twigg, J. and Atkin, K. (1991) *Evaluating Support to Informal Carers (Part 2)*, DSS 809, Social Policy Research Unit, University of York.

Twigg, J. and Atkin, K. with Perring, C. (1990a) *Carers and Services: A Review of Research*, London, HMSO.

Twigg, J., Atkin, K. and Perring, C. (1990b) *Evaluating Support to Informal Carers (Part 1)*, DSS 709, Social Policy Research Unit, University of York.

Ungerson, C. (1983) Women and caring: skills, tasks and taboos, in *The Public and the Private*, edited by Gamarnikow, D., Morgan, D., Purvis, J. and Taylorson, D., London, Heinemann.

Ungerson, C. (1987) *Policy is Personal: Sex, Gender and Informal Care*, London, Tavistock.

Ungerson, C. (ed.) (1991) *Gender and Caring; Work and Welfare in Britain and Scandinavia*, Hemel Hempstead, Wheatsheaf.

Ungerson, C. and Baldock, J. (1991) What d'ya want if you don' want money? – a feminist critique of paid volunteering, in *Women's Issues in Social Policy*, edited by Maclean, M. and Groves, D., London, Routledge.

Ungerson, C. (forthcoming) Payment for caring: mapping a territory, in *The Costs of Welfare*, edited by Deakin, N. and Page, R., Aldershot, Avebury.

Vaughn, C.E. and Leff, J.P. (1976) The influence of family and social factors on the course of psychiatric illness: a comparison of schizophrenic and depressed neurotic patients, *British Journal of Psychiatry*, 129.

Vaugh, C.E. and Leff, J.P. (1981) Patterns of emotional response in relatives of schizophrenic patients, *Schizophrenia Bulletin*, 7(1).

Waerness, K. (1984) The rationality of caring, *Economic and Industrial Democracy*, 5.

Walker, A. (ed.) (1982) *Community Care: The Family, the State and Social Policy*, Oxford, Blackwell and Robertson.

Warburton, W. (1988) *Key Indicators of Local Authority Social Services: A Demonstration Package*, London, Social Services Inspectorate, Department of Health and Social Security.

Ward, L. (1990) A programme for change: current issues in services for people with learning disabilities, in *Better Lives: Changing Services for People with Learning Difficulties*, edited by Booth, T., Sheffield, Joint Unit for Social Services Research/Community Care.

Webb, A. and Wistow, G. (1982) *Whither State Welfare? Policy and Implementation in the Personal Social Services 1979–80*, London, Royal Institute of Public Administration.

Welsh Office (1983) *All Wales Strategy for the Development of Services for Mentally Handicapped People*, London, HMSO.

Wenger, C. (1984) *The Supportive Network: Coping with Old Age*, London, George Allen and Unwin.

Wertheimer, A. (1989) *Housing, the Foundation of Community Care*, London, NFHA and MIND.

West, P., Illsley, R. and Kelman, H. (1984) Public preferences for the care of dependency groups, *Social Science and Medicine*, 18.

Wicks, M. (1982) Community care and elderly people, in *Community Care: The Family, the State and Social Policy*, edited by Walker, A., Oxford, Blackwell and Robertson.

Wildavsky, A. (1979) *Speaking Truth to Power: the Art and Craft Policy Analysis*, Boston, Little Brown.

Williams, F. (1989) *Social Policy: A Critical Introduction*, London, Polity Press.

Wilson, E. (1982) Women, the 'community' and the 'family', in *Community Care: The Family and Social Policy*, edited by Walker, A., Oxford, Blackwell.

Wolfensberger, W. and Thomas, S. (1985) *Program Analysis of Service Systems: Implementation of Normalisation Goals*, Toronto, National Institute of Mental Retardation.

Wright, F.D. (1986) *Left to Care Alone*, Aldershot, Gower.

Wright, K. (1987) *The Economics of Informal Care of the Elderly*, Discussion Paper 23, Centre for Health Economics, University of York.

Young, M. and Wilmot, P. (1957) *Family and Kinship in East London*, London, Routledge and Kegan Paul.

Zarit, S.H. (1989) Do we need another 'stress and caregiving' study?, *Gerontologist*, 29(2).

INDEX

THE FUTURE FOR PALLIATIVE CARE
ISSUES OF POLICY AND PRACTICE

David Clark (ed.)

In recent years the independent hospice movement has done a great deal to promote care standards. But many issues remain unresolved. Can and should the hospice approach be translated into other settings? How can care be improved in hospitals, in the community, and in residential and nursing homes? How can such care be costed and evaluated? What new service initiatives are required and how are these affected by changes in government policy? How do planners and practitioners address the ethical and cultural needs of a changing society?

Drawing on a variety of disciplines and specialties in medicine, nursing and the social sciences, expert contributors explore the future for palliative care, paying particular attention to the relationship between policy and practice.

This challenging volume breaks new ground in our thinking about how dying people should be cared for and will be essential reading for practitioners, students and researchers in palliative care.

Contents
Introduction – Where and how people die – Quality, costs and contracts of care – Informal care and community care – Developments in bereavement services – HIV/AIDS: lessons for policy and practice – Cultural issues in terminal care – Euthanasia – The medicalization of dying – A doctor's view – Issues in pain management – Whither the hospices? – Index.

Contributors
Sam Ahmedzai, Richard Atkinson, Bronwen Biswas, David Clark, Tony Crowther, Graham Davies, Ann Faulkner, David Field, Shirley Firth, Barry Hancock, Irene Higginson, Nicky James, Brenda Neale, Neil Small, Eric Wilkes.

192pp 0 335 15764 5 (Paperback) 0 335 15765 3 (Hardbook)

COORDINATING COMMUNITY CARE
MULTIDISCIPLINARY TEAMS AND CARE MANAGEMENT

John Øvretveit

This book is about how people from different professions and agencies work together to meet the health and social needs of people in a community. It is about making the most of different skills to meet people's needs, and creating satisfying and supportive working groups. It is about the details of making community care a reality.

The effectiveness and quality of care a person receives depends on getting the right professionals and services, and also on the support given to the person's carers. Services must be coordinated if the person is to benefit, but coordination is more difficult with the increasing change, variety and complexity of health and social services in the 1990s. This book challenges the assumptions that services are best coordinated by multi-professional and multi-agency teams, and that community care teams are broadly similar. It demonstrates when a team is needed and how to overcome differences between professions, and between agency policies and philosophies.

Drawing on ten years of consultancy research with a variety of teams and services, the author gives practical guidance for managers and practitioners about how to set up and improve coordination and teamwork. The book combines practical concerns with theoretical depth drawing on organization and management theory, psychology, psychoanalysis, sociology, economics and government studies.

Contents

Introduction – Needs and organization – Markets, bureaucracy and association – Types of team – Client pathways and team resource management – Team members' roles – Team leadership – Decisions and conflict in teams – Communications and co-service – Coordinating community health and social care – Appendices – Glossary – References and bibliography – Index.

240pp   0 335 19047 2 (Paperback)   0 335 19048 0 (Hardback)

CARING FOR PEOPLE
HELP AT THE FRONTLINE

Jenny Rogers

A careworker is in the 'frontline'; is often the person who deals first with clients who are frightened, upset, confused, angry and lonely; who washes, toilets and dresses clients; who sits with a dying client and deals with the bereaved relatives. *Caring for People* provides invaluable and practical guidance for all frontline carers. It discusses how best to empathize with the client, how to listen, assess risks, encourage clients' self esteem and independence. It deals with the routine daily tasks, and how to cope with the emergencies. It shows how to avoid stress in the job, and advises on career development. It is a down to earth handbook for all careworkers.

Contents

176pp 0 335 09429 5 (Paperback) 0 335 09430 9 (Hardback)

WITH THIS BODY
CARING AND DISABILITY IN MARRIAGE

Gillian Parker

This book breaks new ground by examining the views both of younger people who become disabled after marriage and of their partners who become involved in helping and supporting them. It explores the giving and receiving of personal care in marriage, and the roles of informal networks, services and income in supporting these couples and their children. It shows how, in the absence of help and support from elsewhere, couples are left in an extremely precarious position – practically, financially, emotionally, and socially. Disabled people argue the need for resources and services that would allow them to be independent of 'informal' help. This book shows that age, class, gender and existing power relations in the marriage affect the experience of both disability and caring and the extent to which 'independence' from informal help is seen by either partner as a legitimate or desirable goal.

Contents

160pp 0 335 09946 7 (Paperback) 0 335 09947 5 (Hardback)